FOREPLAY

The Art of Stretching for Golf

First edition
Pica La Balle, Inc. • Napa, California

FOREPLAY
The Art of Stretching for Golf

By Patti DeVincenzi
& Suzanne Curtis, P.T.

Published by Pica La Balle, Inc.
Post Office Box 3129
Napa, California 94558

First Printing 1992
Printed in the United States of America

This book is available at special discounts for bulk purchases for sales premiums, fund-raising or educational use. For details contact Special Sales Department, Pica La Balle, Inc.

Library of Congress Catalog Card Number: 92-80538
ISBN 0-9631840-8-3: $19.95 Softcover

PLEASE READ THIS

Readers are strongly cautioned to consult with a physician or other health-care professional *before* engaging in the exercises described in FOREPLAY: THE ART OF STRETCHING FOR GOLF, and to tailor the exercises in the book to meet the reader's special needs.

FOREPLAY: THE ART OF STRETCHING FOR GOLF is based on information obtained from sources believed to be reliable, and every effort has been made to make the book as complete and accurate as possible based on information available as of the printing date, but its accuracy and completeness cannot be guaranteed. Despite the best efforts of author and publisher, the book may contain mistakes, and the reader should use the book only as a general guide and not as the ultimate source of information about golf, exercise or stretching.

The book is not intended to reprint all of the information available to the author or publisher on the subject, but rather to simplify, complement and supplement other available sources. The reader is encouraged to read all available material and to learn as much possible about the subject. Some of these materials are listed under SUGGESTED READING on page 34.

The author and the publisher are not engaged in rendering medical services, and the book is not intended to diagnose or treat medical or physical problems. If medical, professional or other expert assistance is required by the reader, please seek the services of a competent expert.

FOREPLAY is sold without warranties of any kind, express or implied, and Pica La Balle, Inc. and the author disclaim any liability, loss or damage caused by the information contained in this book.

IF YOU DO NOT WISH TO BE BOUND BY THE FOREGOING CAUTIONS AND CONDITIONS, YOU MAY RETURN THE BOOK TO THE PUBLISHER FOR A FULL REFUND.

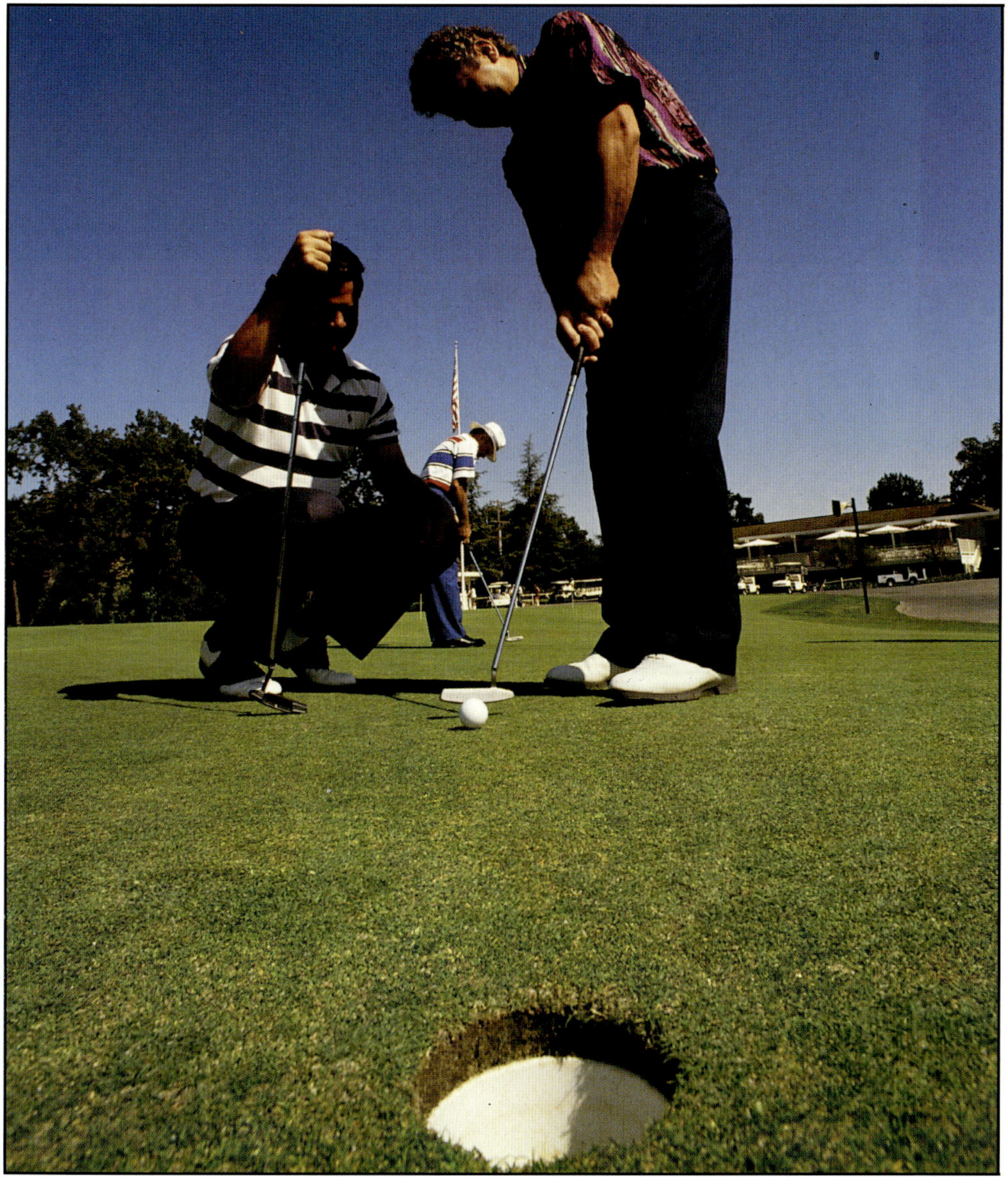

SPECIAL THANKS TO:

SILVERADO COUNTRY CLUB &
RESORT * Napa, California

Brian Curtis, P.T.
Jeff Goodwin, Golf Professional
Kirk Candland
Bert & Elke Grobs
Mel Valdez
David West
Jimmy Ballard, Golf Professional
Marty James, Sports Editor
Robert Muir Graves,
Golf Course Architect
Dr. Gary Wiren,
PGA Master Professional
Jim Clover, A.T.C.
Tom Lorren, P.T.
Stephen Hochschuler, M.D.
Janice Capobianco, P.T.
Rolla D. Campbell, Jr., M.D.
Robert J. Albo, M.D.
Robert Galley, M.S.Ed., P.T.

Photography by:
Bruce Evensen, M.Photg.Cr.

> *"Flexibility is critical to golf performance. Without it, having strength alone, would be like having a powerful auto engine without an adequate transmission to get the force to the wheels."*
> — Dr. Gary Wiren, PGA Master Professional

The sole purpose of *FOREPLAY* is to help you improve your flexibility for the sport of golf.

I discovered that I could wisely spend the idle time waiting for the first tee or waiting for the green to clear by doing some simple, effective stretching. Constant, nagging lower back pain and the realization that precious time on the golf course was being wasted motivated me to be instructed on a warm-up program that could be done anytime or anywhere. Stretching activities are not yet typically seen on the golf course and I have found most people are quite curious and highly interested in learning about a professionally designed warm-up routine. Until now, only a fortunate few have been able to enjoy a program like this. *FOREPLAY* gives you the inside track on stretching for golf. We introduce just one aspect of an overall golf program that should include flexibility, strengthening, cardiovascular conditioning and regular visits to your golf professional. In this book you will find a program that can be done under ideal conditions, such as in the home at your leisure. You can also abbreviate this program for a hurry-up when you are running late or for a dewy/frosty day. A handy travel card is included so you can remember your program. In the future most golf courses will probably provide a stretch area in or around the clubhouse where you'll be able to do your pre-game warm-up routine (including floor and upright stretches) under perfect conditions; until then you must improvise.

More frequently we are hearing golf commentators on T.V. talk about professional golfers bad backs and how sports medicine experts stand ready for their individualized treatments. Follow the tips found in this book and you will have your own individualized program too! Pro golfers experience the tremendous benefits of proper warm-up and these are things that the regular golf consumer must also demand.

Did you know that it is equally important to be trained by an expert in proper body mechanics as it is to be trained by an expert in proper golf fundamentals? Therefore, you will want to consult your health care professional for a general physical and most importantly get a referral for a sports medicine specialist, such as a physical therapist, for training on proper body mechanics. The benefit of this experience, apart from the obvious, includes your own personalized program that will factor in your personal lifestyle and you'll find out how to prevent injuries that can result from golf activities. We know that certain activities combining bending, reaching and turning can cause big problems. This might include taking clubs from your trunk, stooping to take the ball from the hole, riding in golf carts or just plain clunking the shot. Believe me, if you love golf as much as I do, you will want to do everything you can to play injury free. The same philosophy holds true with cars as with health, it's cheaper to have regular maintenance done than to have to fix a catastrophe. Remember, PREVENTION IS THE BEST MEDICINE.

This book, combined with your individualized program will give you a systematic blueprint to follow every day. The hard part is getting started, but once you feel the difference you'll find yourself stretching automatically. Why wait another day to experience the benefits of a stretching program when it may be the one thing that gives you the competitive advantage?

Together we can make the practice of proper warm-up at the first tee acceptable and routine for every golfer. We'll wonder why we waited so long to make this great event a priority in our golf game.

As always, visit your resident PGA Golf Professional as much as possible for technical expertise on the game of golf.

Pica la Balle Bene - Hit the ball well!

Patti DeVincenzi

WHY STRETCH FOR GOLF

Stretching will:

- Reduce your chances of minor injury
- Increase range of motion
- Elongate your soft tissues

Faithful stretching and devoted practicing, coupled with the counsel of your PGA Golf Professional, all have a part in perfecting form and injury prevention.

WHEN TO STRETCH FOR GOLF

Stretch after warming up the large muscle groups, before your first swing, throughout the game of golf, after the game or whenever you can. Stretching should be done daily regardless of your golf schedule.

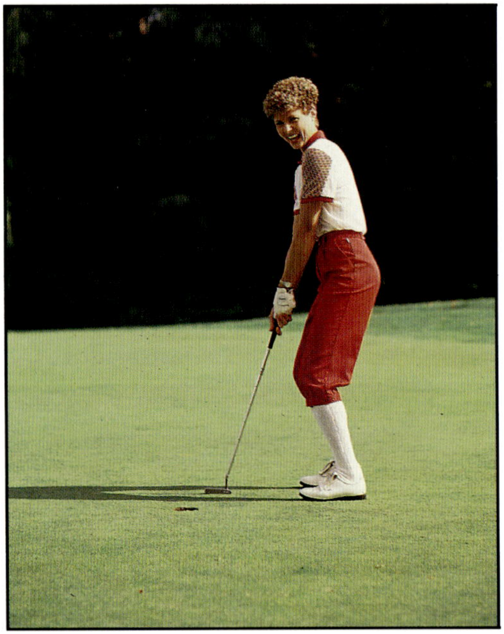

STRETCH GUIDELINES

Start with a few minutes of brisk walking or light jogging immediately before you begin to stretch. Increasing the body's temperature with a brisk walk or light jog immediately before your pre-game stretching allows you to stretch more effectively.

Slowly ease into each stretch, without bouncing.

Relax while concentrating on the areas being stretched. Breathe regularly.

Hold the stretch for up to one minute. Generally, beginners should hold 10-20 seconds, others 10-60 seconds. Good common sense should be used in learning duration and distance of stretch. Although longer is better, any FOREPLAY is better than none.

One thing we do know is YOUR program should be tailored to YOUR personal needs, everyone will have a unique program.

Don't over stretch.

Obviously, if you get dizzy or feel pain, stop.

While holding the stretch you should feel the tension decrease. If it does not, ease off. Gradually begin again until you feel a strong but comfortable stretch.

Never stretch to the point of pain.

Do not bounce.

Do each of the following stretches for 2 repetitions on each side of your body, before you begin to play, and throughout your game if you like. Try to do your program at least five days a week whether you are playing or not. That way you'll be ready to go if someone calls and says "We have an opening for a fourth player in ten minutes! Can you make it?"

LARGE MUSCLE WARM UP

Brisk walking sends oxygen to the body tissue, lubricates the joints and prepares the muscles for the next step of warm up. Walking also can reduce tension and help you relax and feel good.

A brisk walk is ideal for warming up. You should be able to carry on a conversation without difficulty in breathing. Try to walk briskly for 10-30 minutes.

During your consultation with your fitness expert, you will have determined your exercise heart rate. (It's kind of like a tachometer on your car.) Use that information to make sure you are maximizing your experience in this very important part of the program.

Marching in place or a light jog can be substituted for a brisk walk. If you're running late, at least try a few minutes of marching in place.

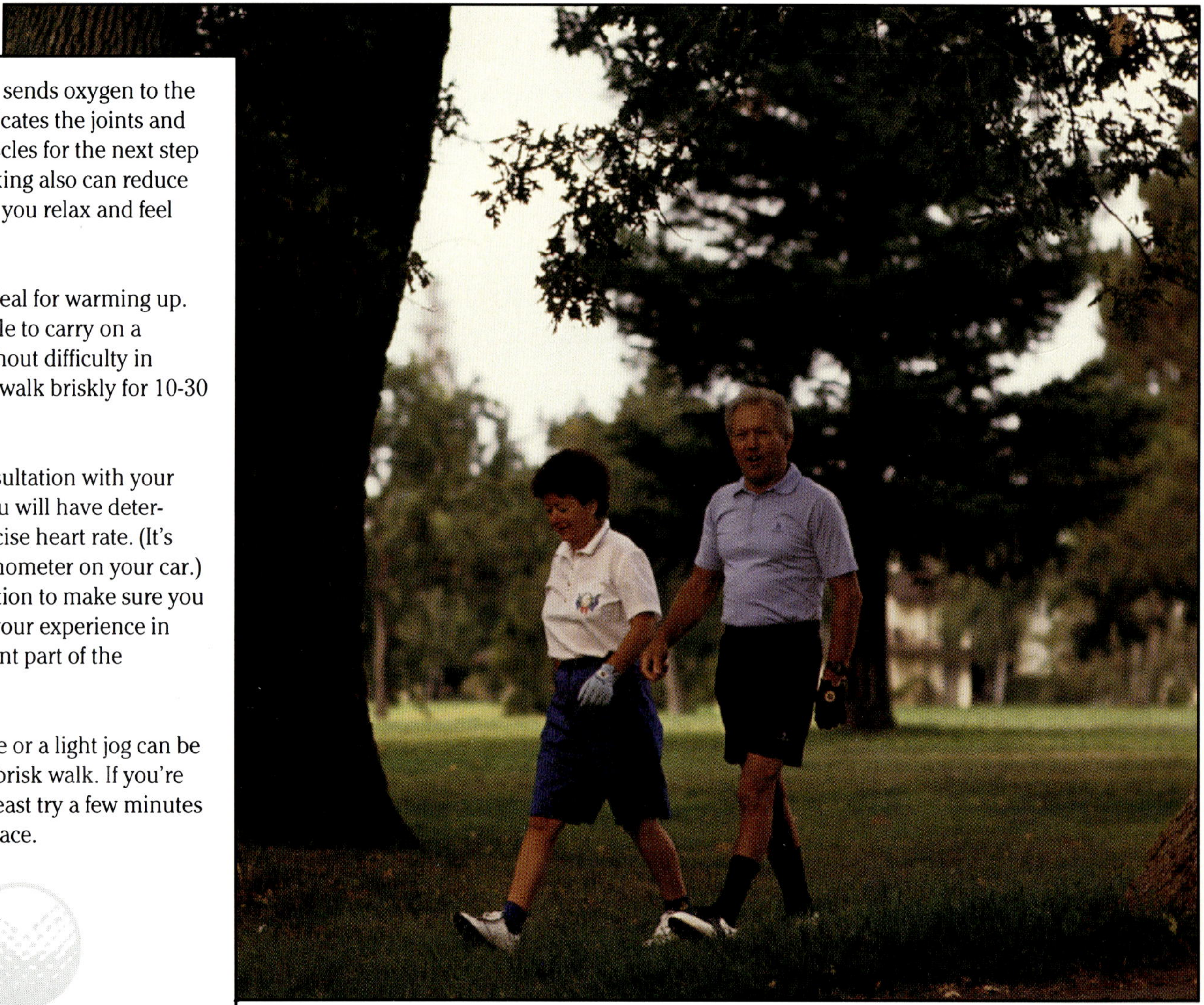

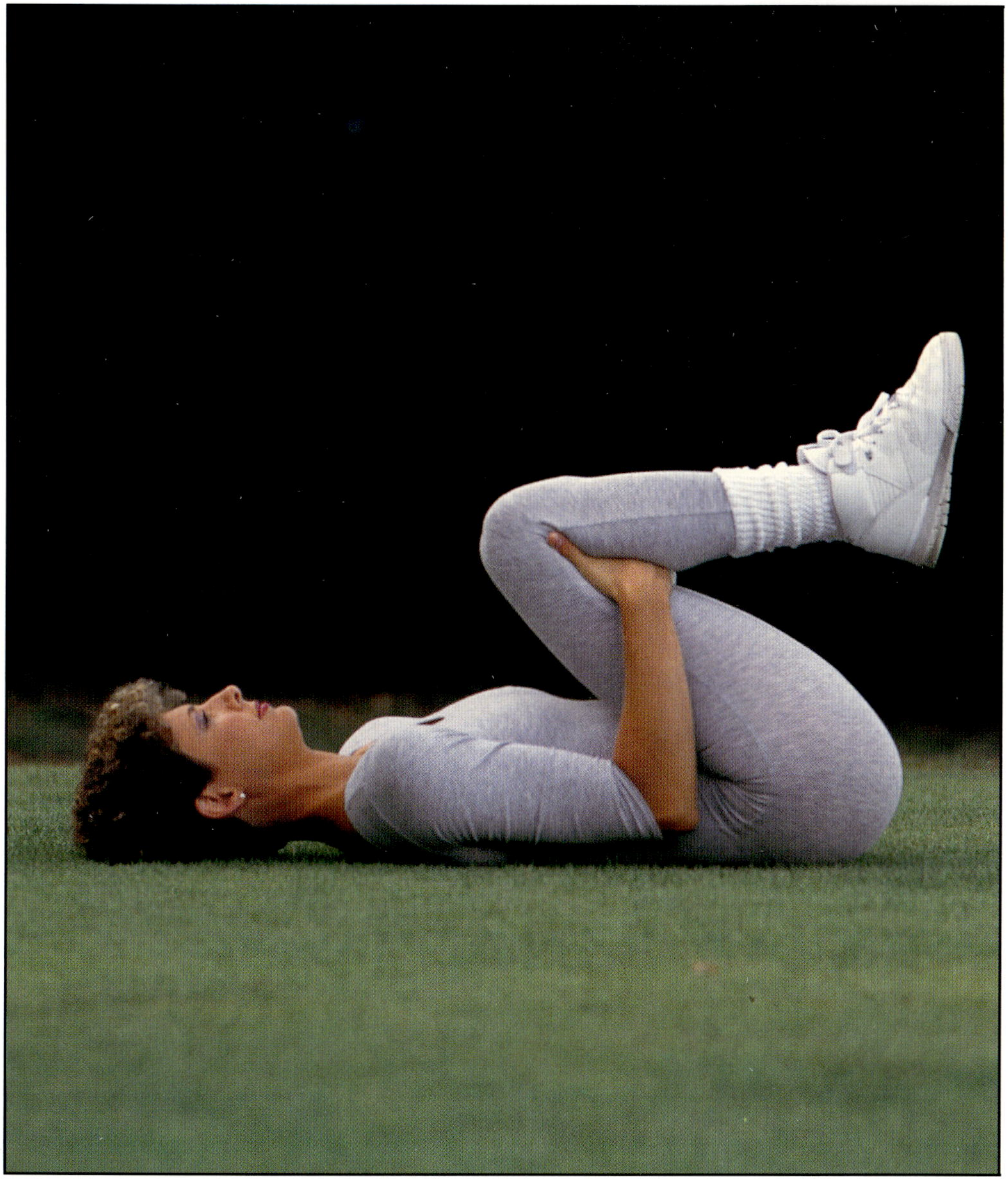

While lying on your back, GENTLY pull your knees toward your chest. Repeat 2 times.

TRUNK and HIP STRETCH

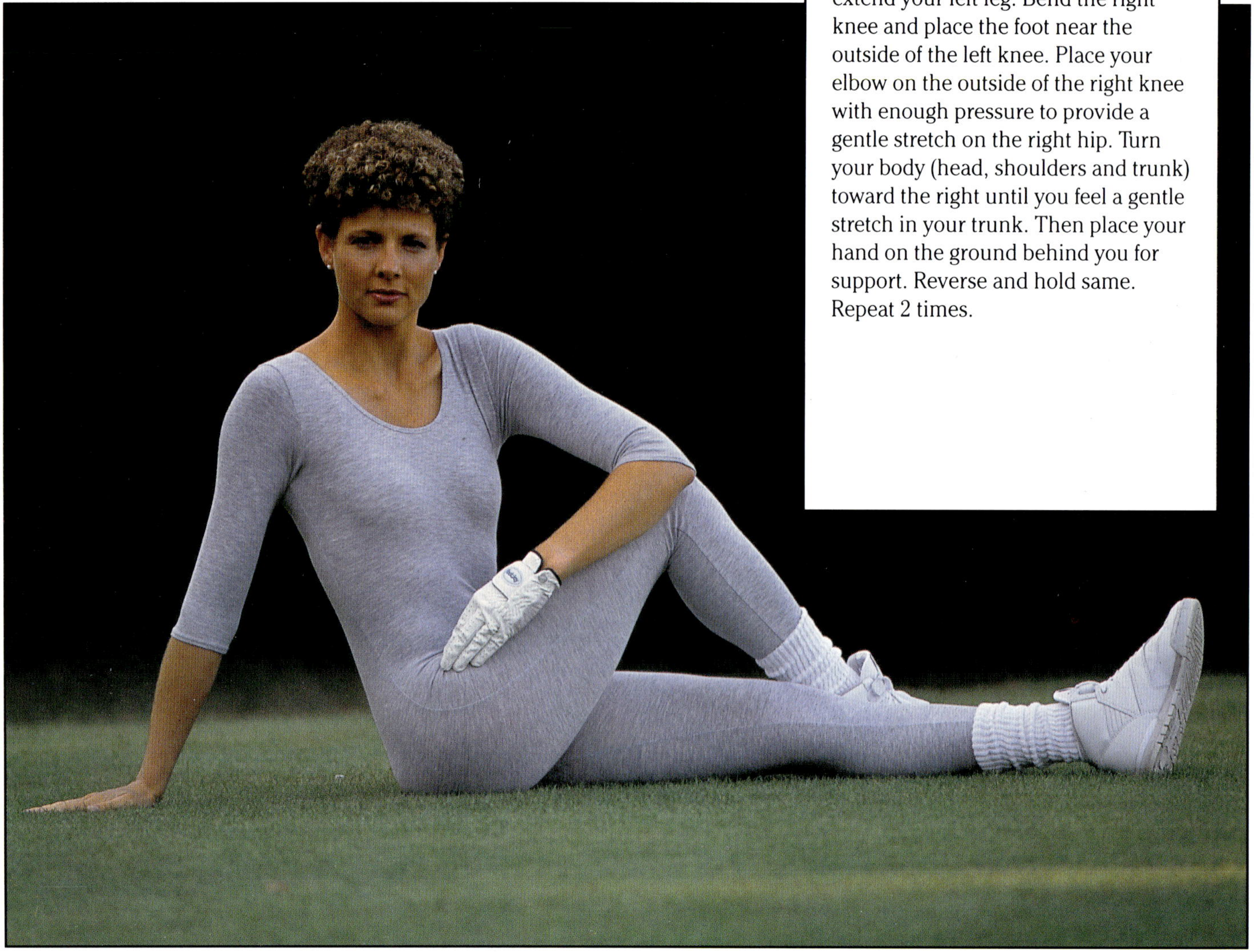

While sitting on the ground, extend your left leg. Bend the right knee and place the foot near the outside of the left knee. Place your elbow on the outside of the right knee with enough pressure to provide a gentle stretch on the right hip. Turn your body (head, shoulders and trunk) toward the right until you feel a gentle stretch in your trunk. Then place your hand on the ground behind you for support. Reverse and hold same. Repeat 2 times.

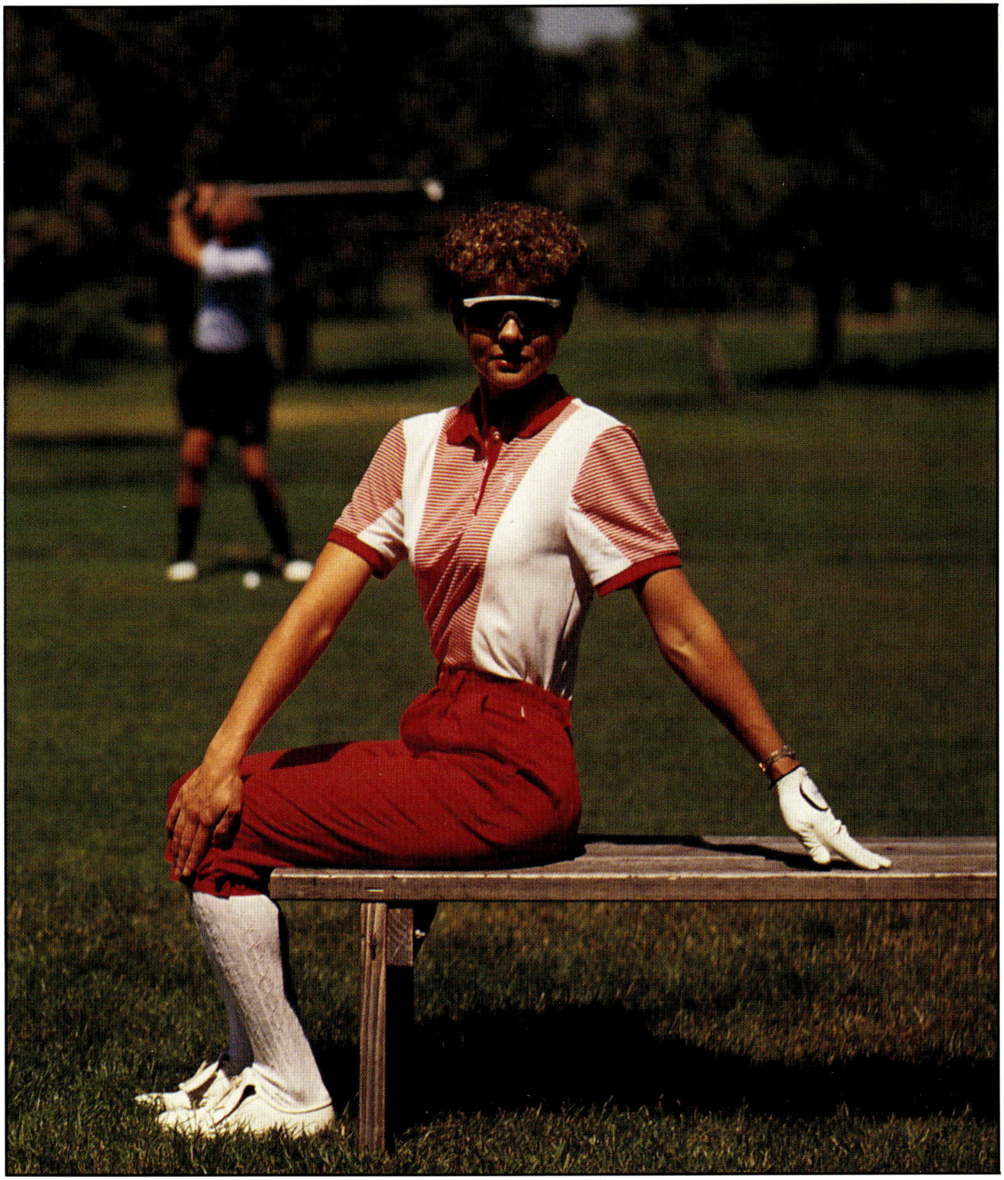

While sitting, reach your right hand to the outside of the left knee. Rotate body until you feel a gentle trunk stretch. Then place your left hand on the bench for support. Reverse and hold same. Repeat 2 times.

TRUNK EXTENSION

Lie down on your stomach. Gently raise up to rest on your elbows and forearms. Let your stomach and hips relax onto the floor. Look straight ahead. Repeat 2 times.

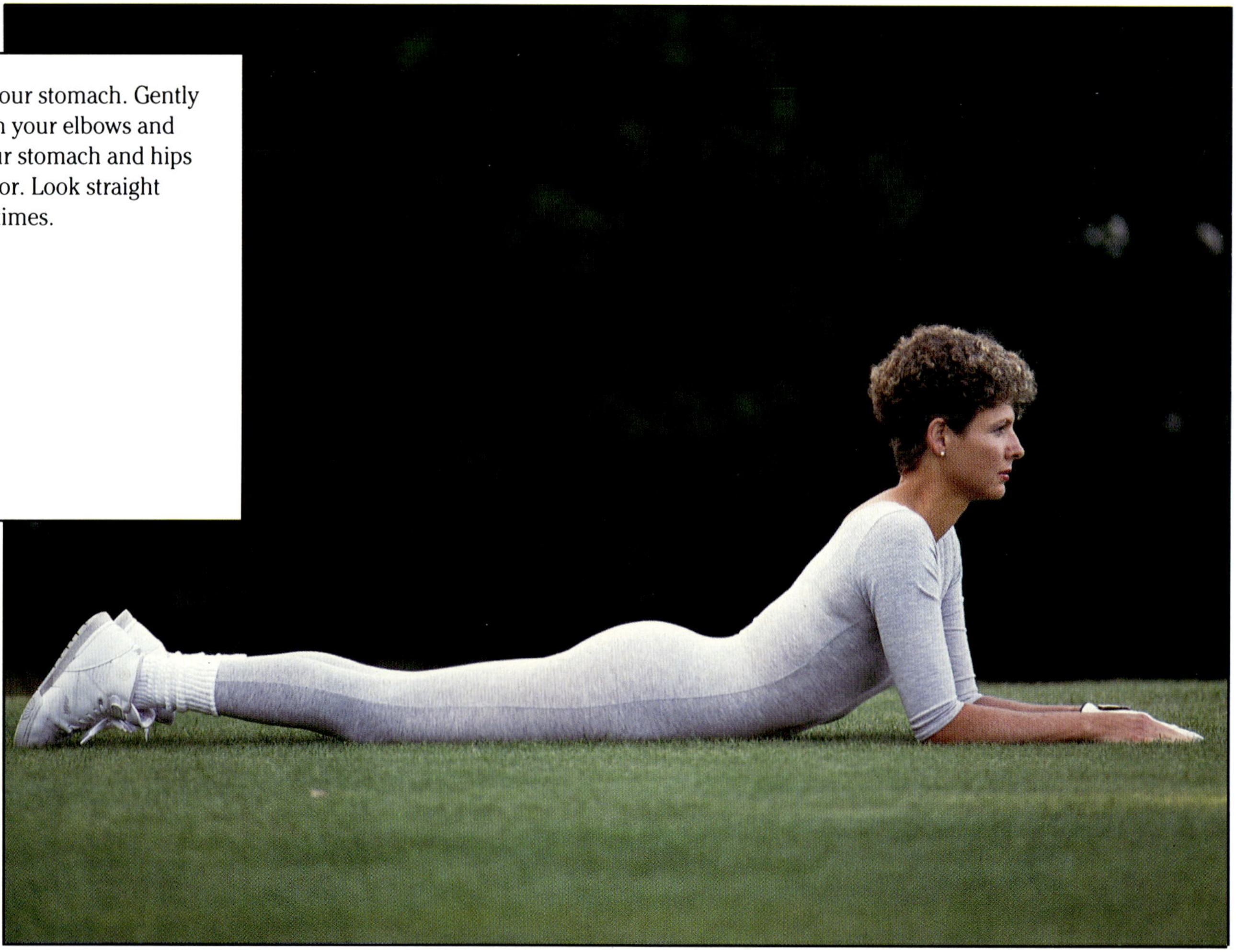

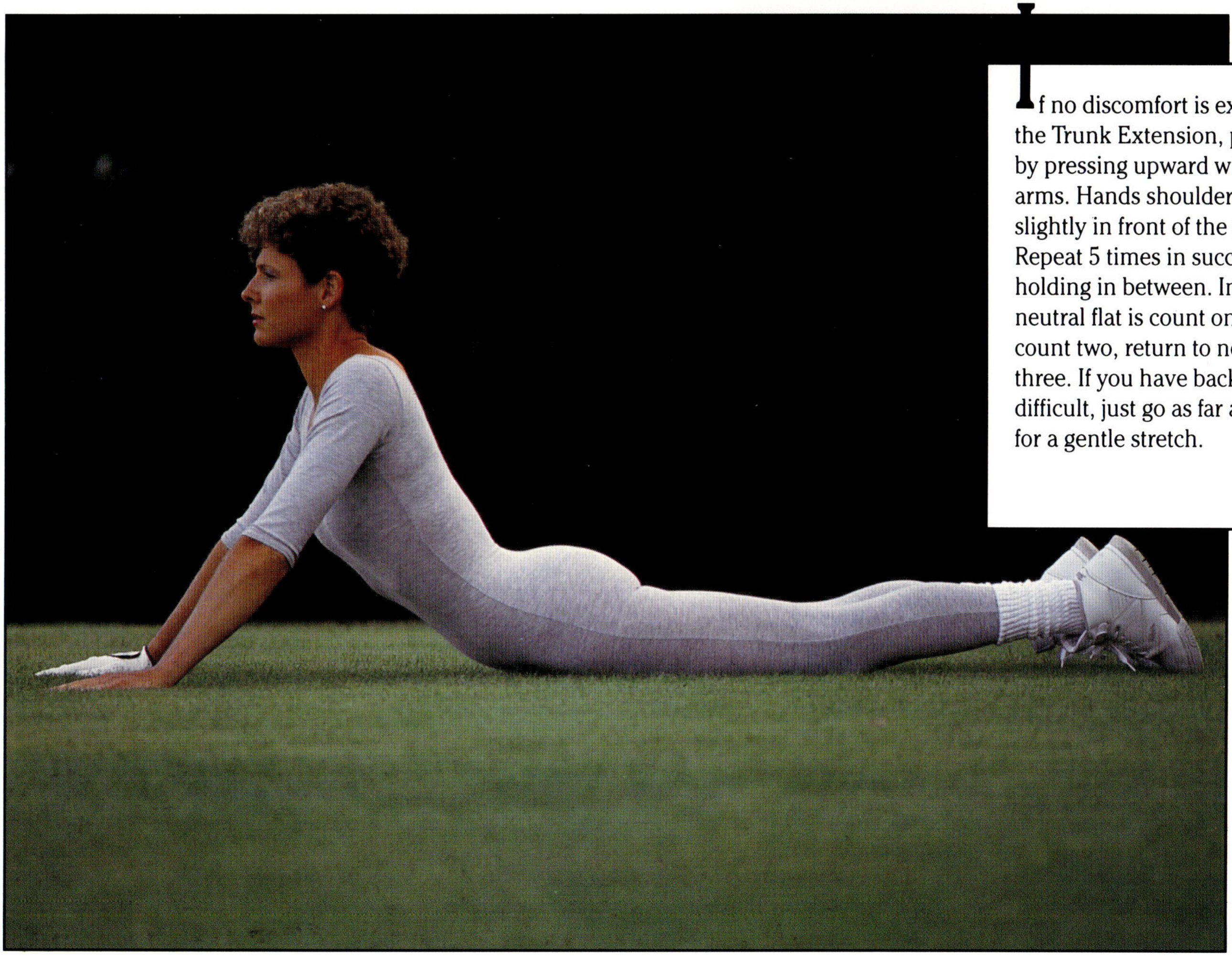

If no discomfort is experienced with the Trunk Extension, progress further by pressing upward with extended arms. Hands shoulder width apart and slightly in front of the shoulders. Repeat 5 times in succession without holding in between. In other words, neutral flat is count one, press up is count two, return to neutral is count three. If you have back pain, or if it is difficult, just go as far as comfortable for a gentle stretch.

UPRIGHT EXTENSION

While standing upright, place hands on lower back. Carefully and slowly lean back as far as is comfortable. Return to the original standing posture. This exercise held for one half count, then return to neutral. Repeat 2 times.

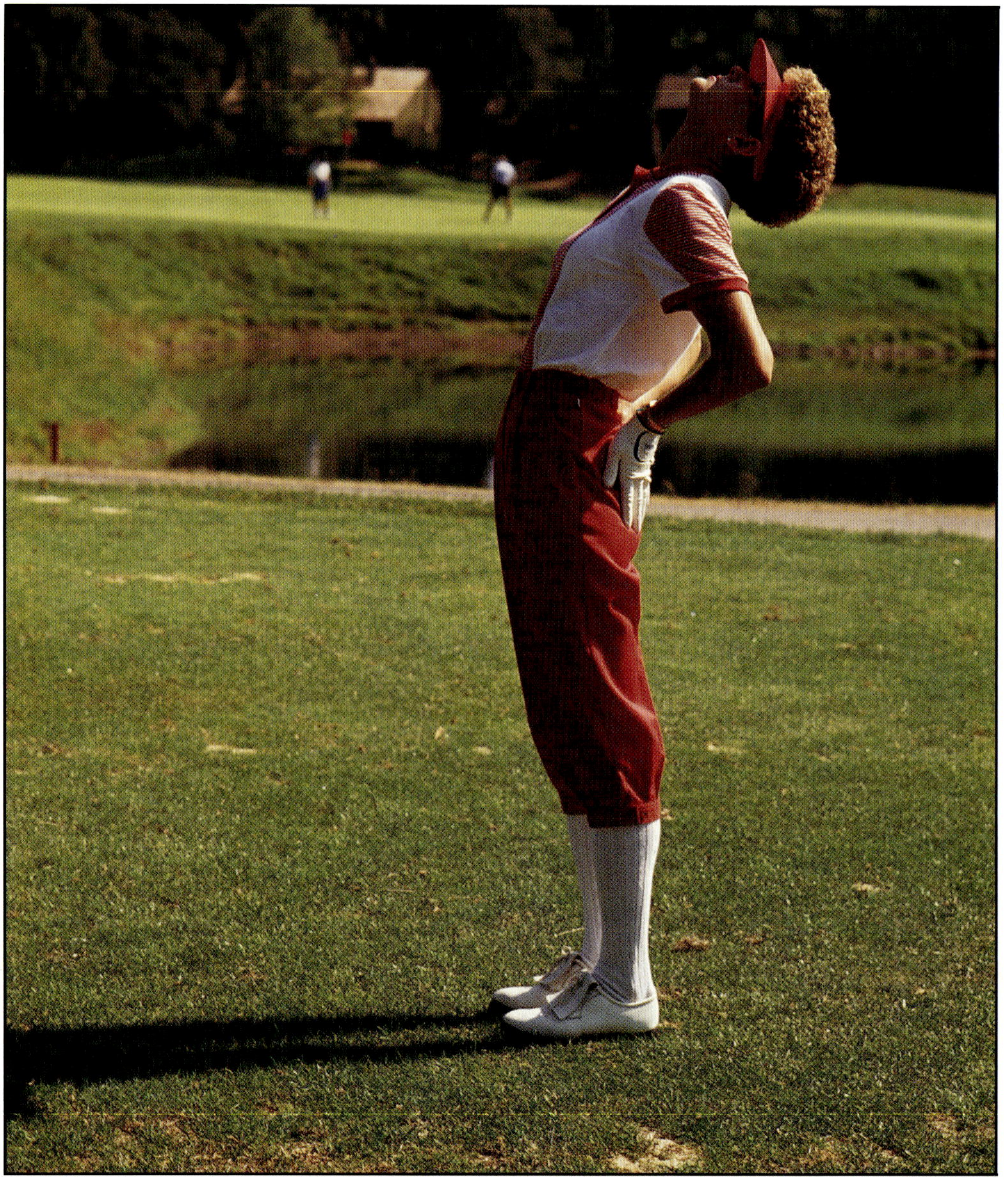

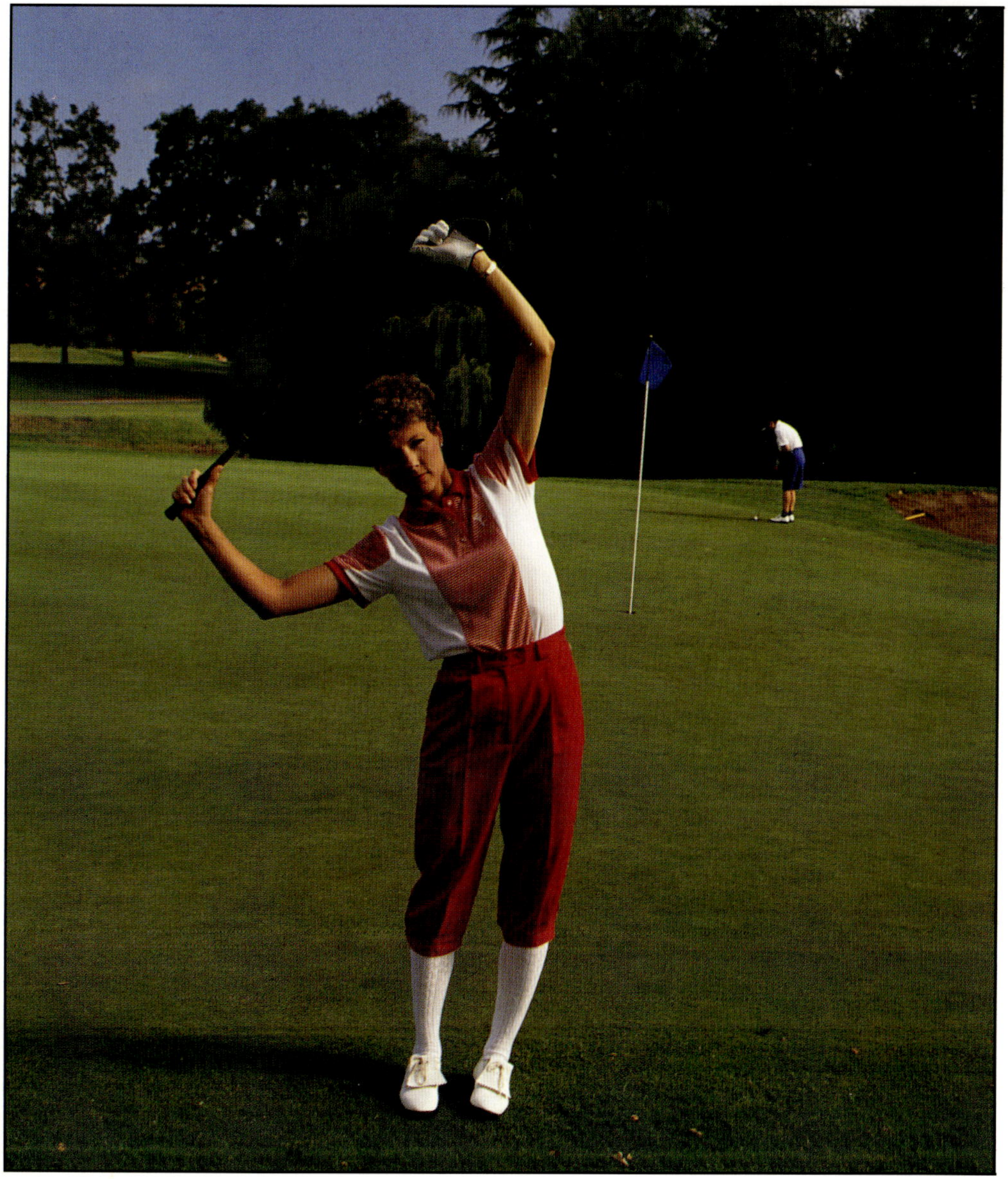

While standing upright, hold a golf club at each end and gently lean to one side and hold, return to neutral and pause, then gently lean to the other side and hold. Repeat 2 times each side.

UPPER ARM AND SHOULDER STRETCH

While standing upright, reach overhead. Grab onto left elbow with right hand. Pull the elbow toward the back of your head. This produces a gentle stretch in the upper arm and trunk. Repeat 2 times on each side.

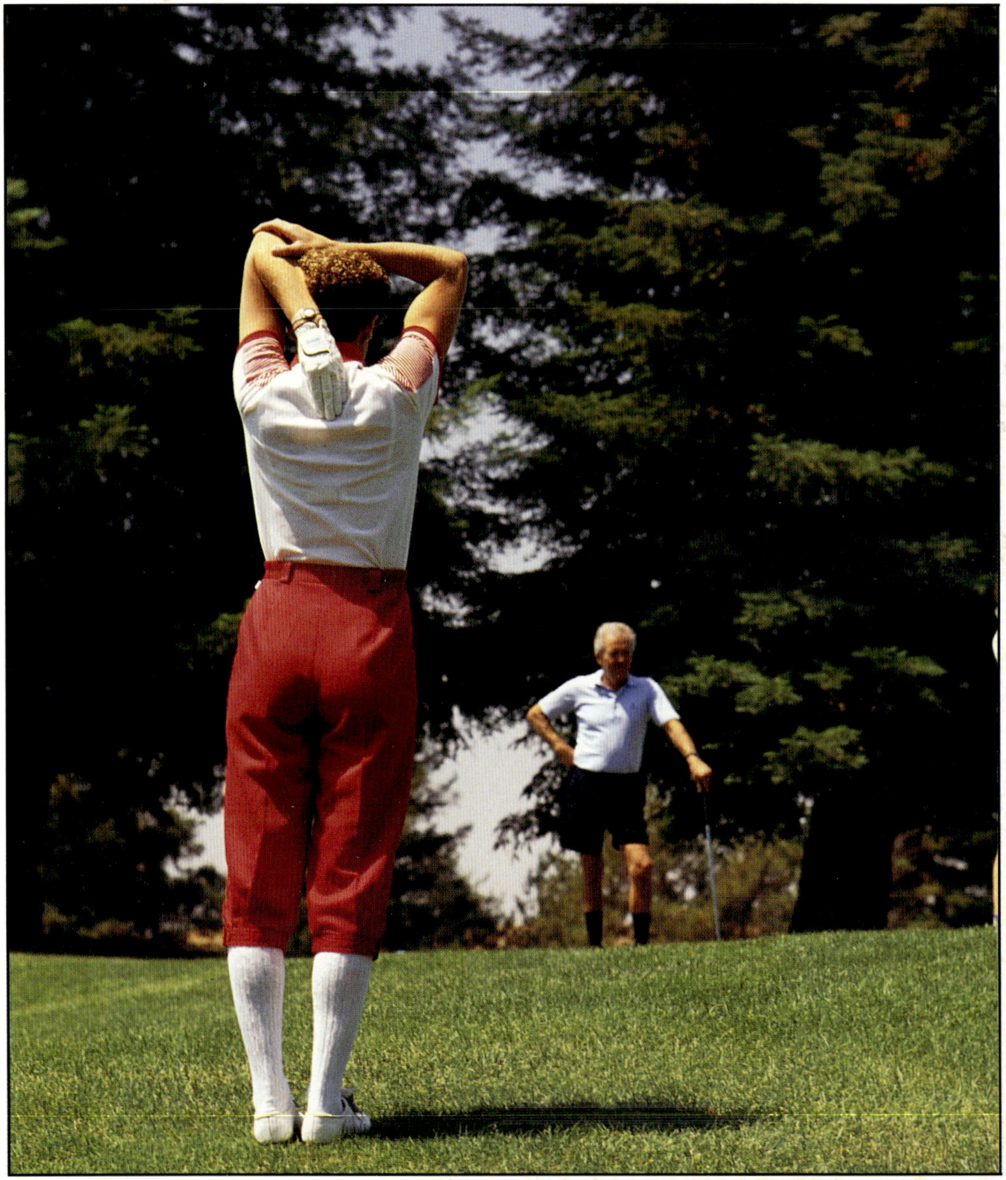

SHOULDER STRETCH

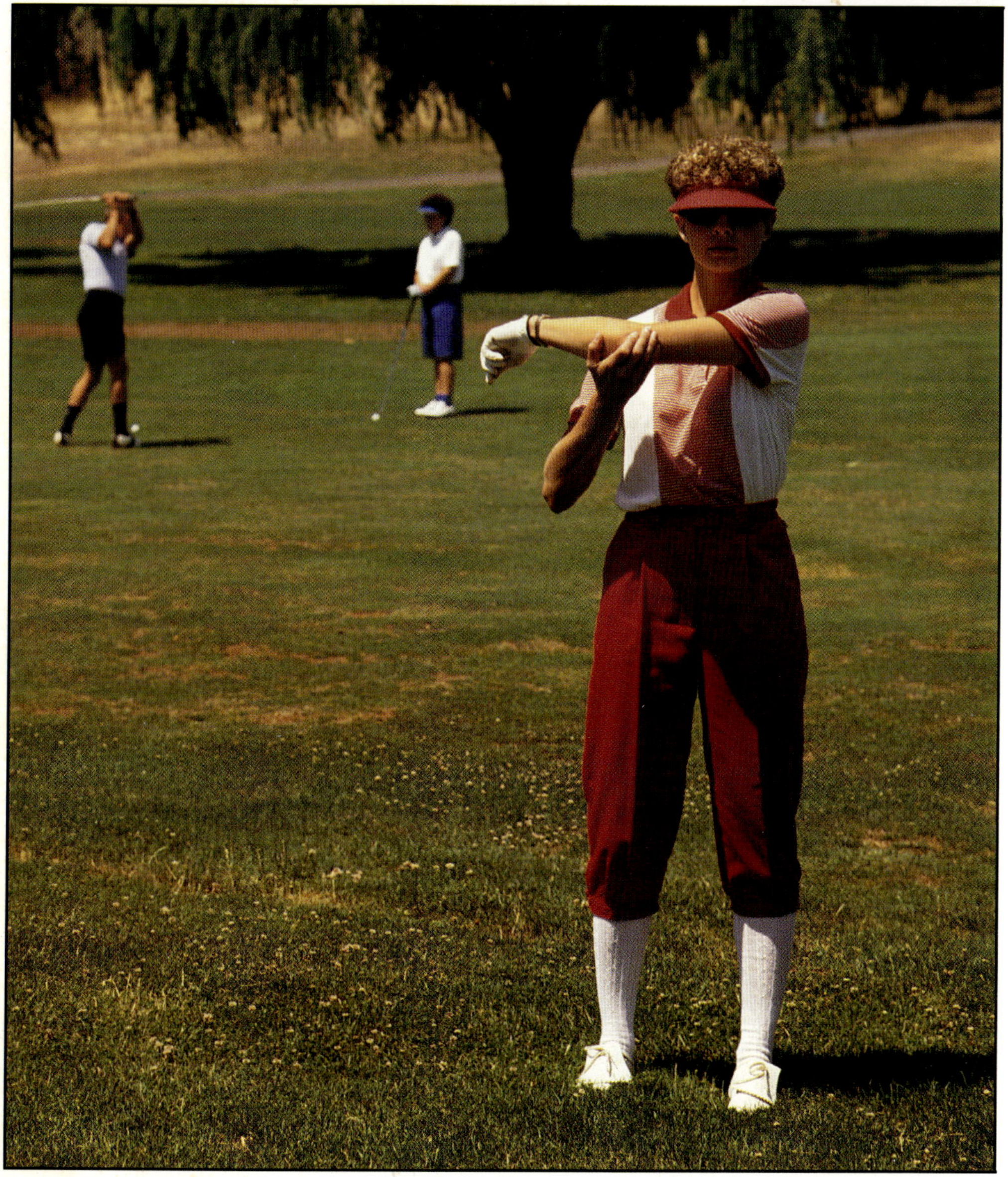

While standing upright, reach across chest and pull your left elbow toward body until a gentle stretch is felt in the upper left back and shoulder region. Repeat 2 times on each side.

CHEST STRETCH

While standing in a doorway, lift arms out to the sides. With elbows cocked allow forearms to rest against the door frame on each side. Hold trunk erect but not arched by contracting stomach and buttocks muscles. Slowly lean forward. Feel a stretch across the chest. Repeat 2 times.

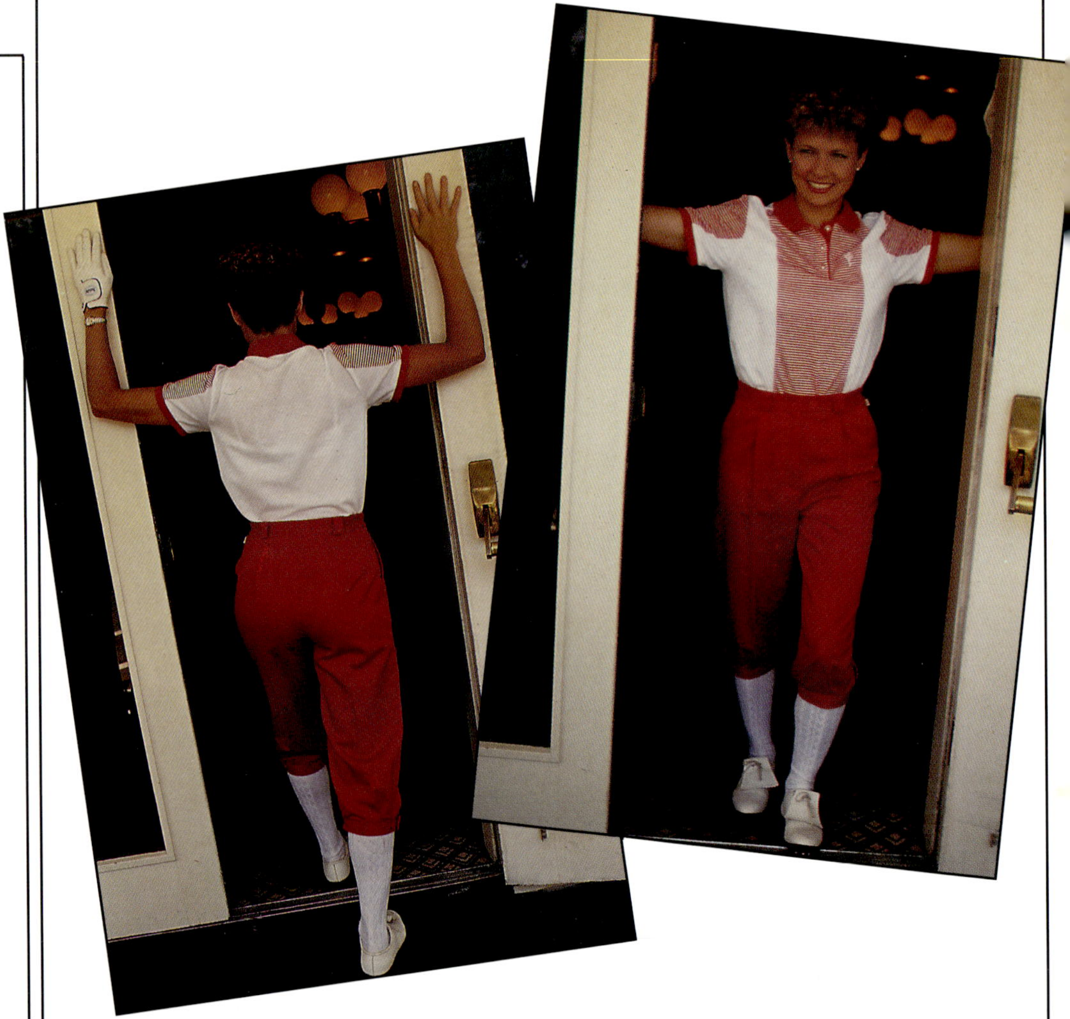

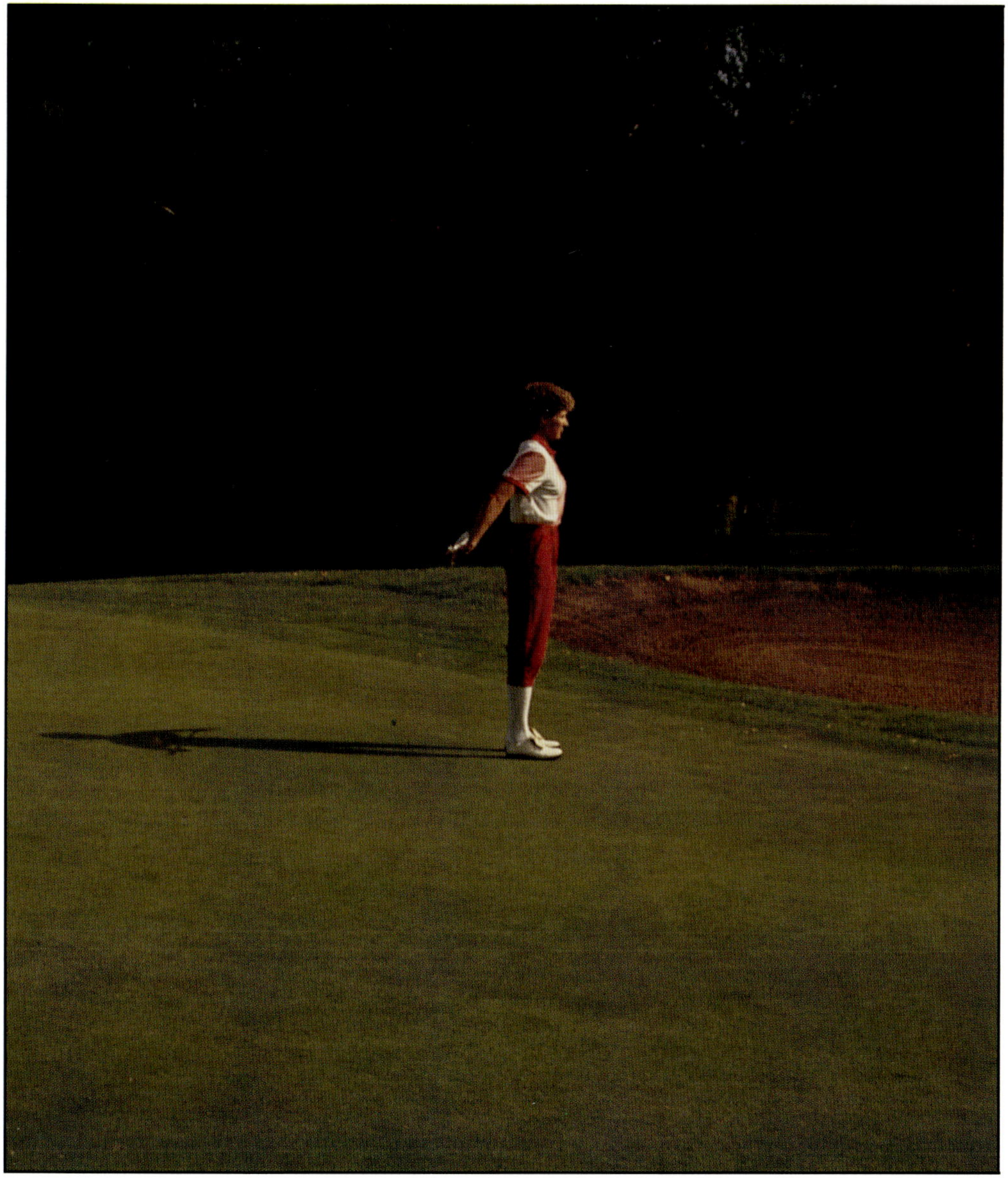

While standing upright, grasp both hands or a golf club behind your back. Pull up and away from your body. Feel a gradual stretch. Avoid leaning forward. Repeat 2 times.

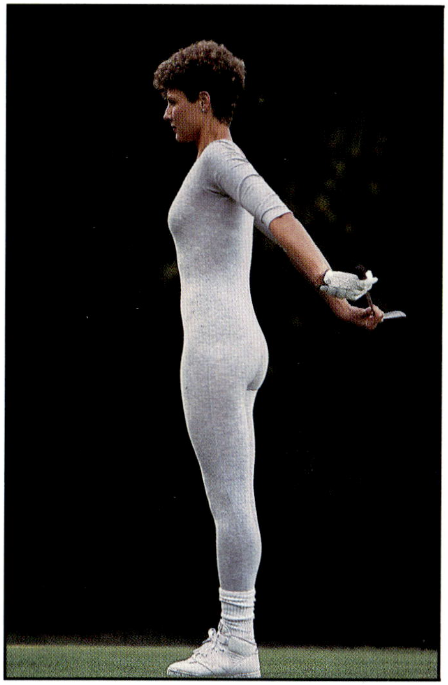

NECK STRETCH - Down

While standing upright, tuck chin into neck and look downward. Head is bent forward. Repeat the neck series 2 times.

Advanced - Very gently apply pressure with your hand.

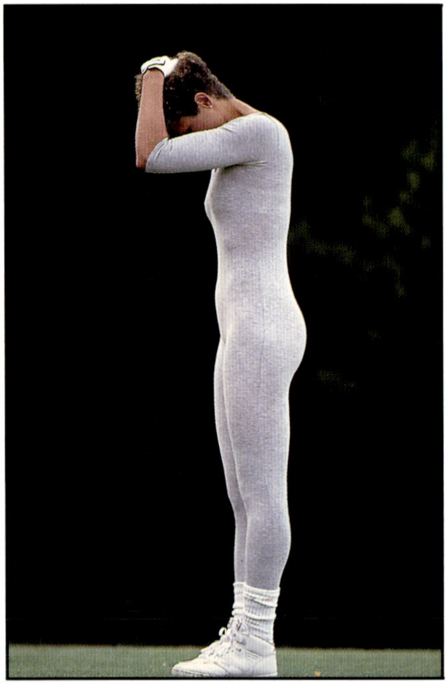

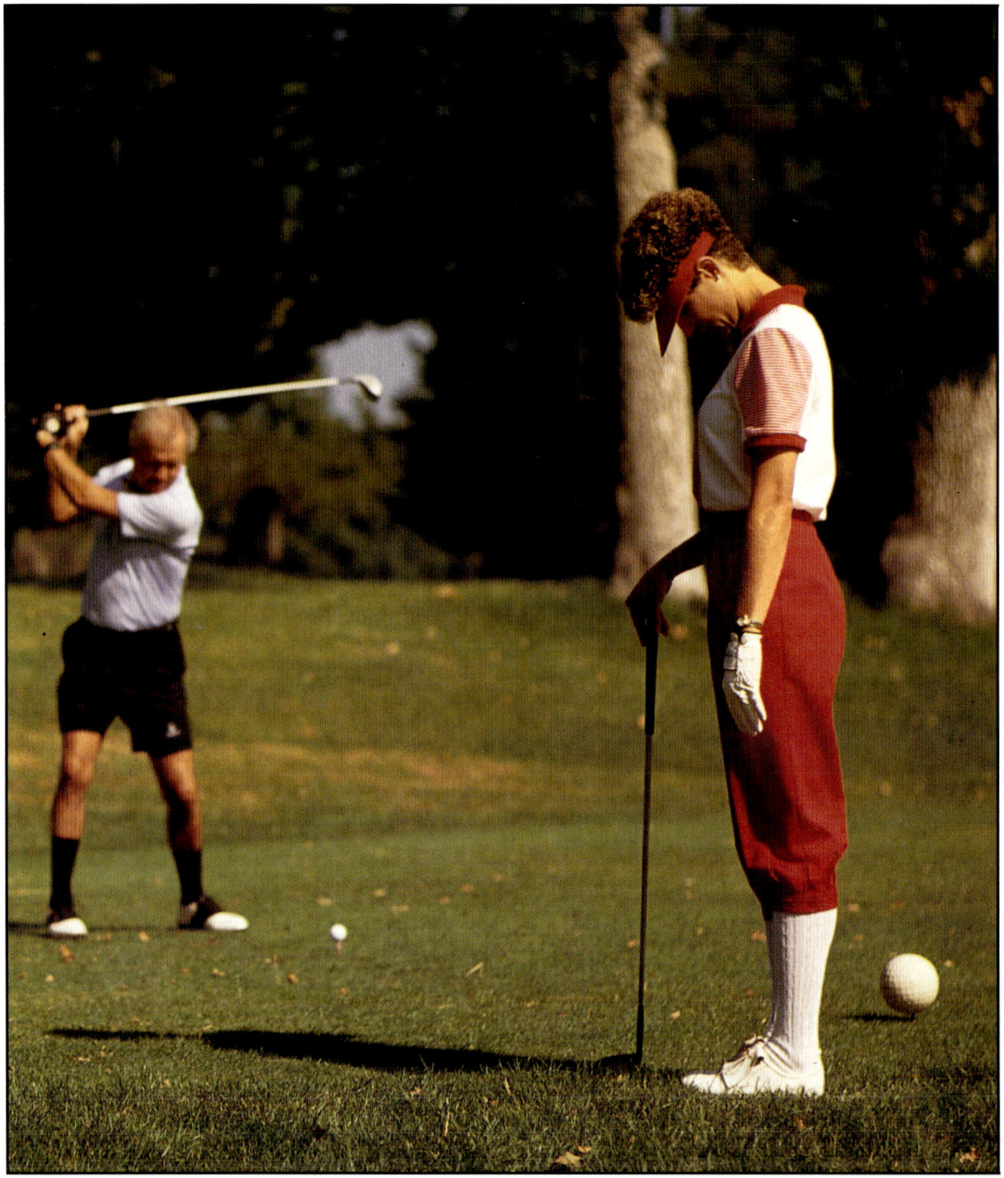

NECK STRETCH - Up

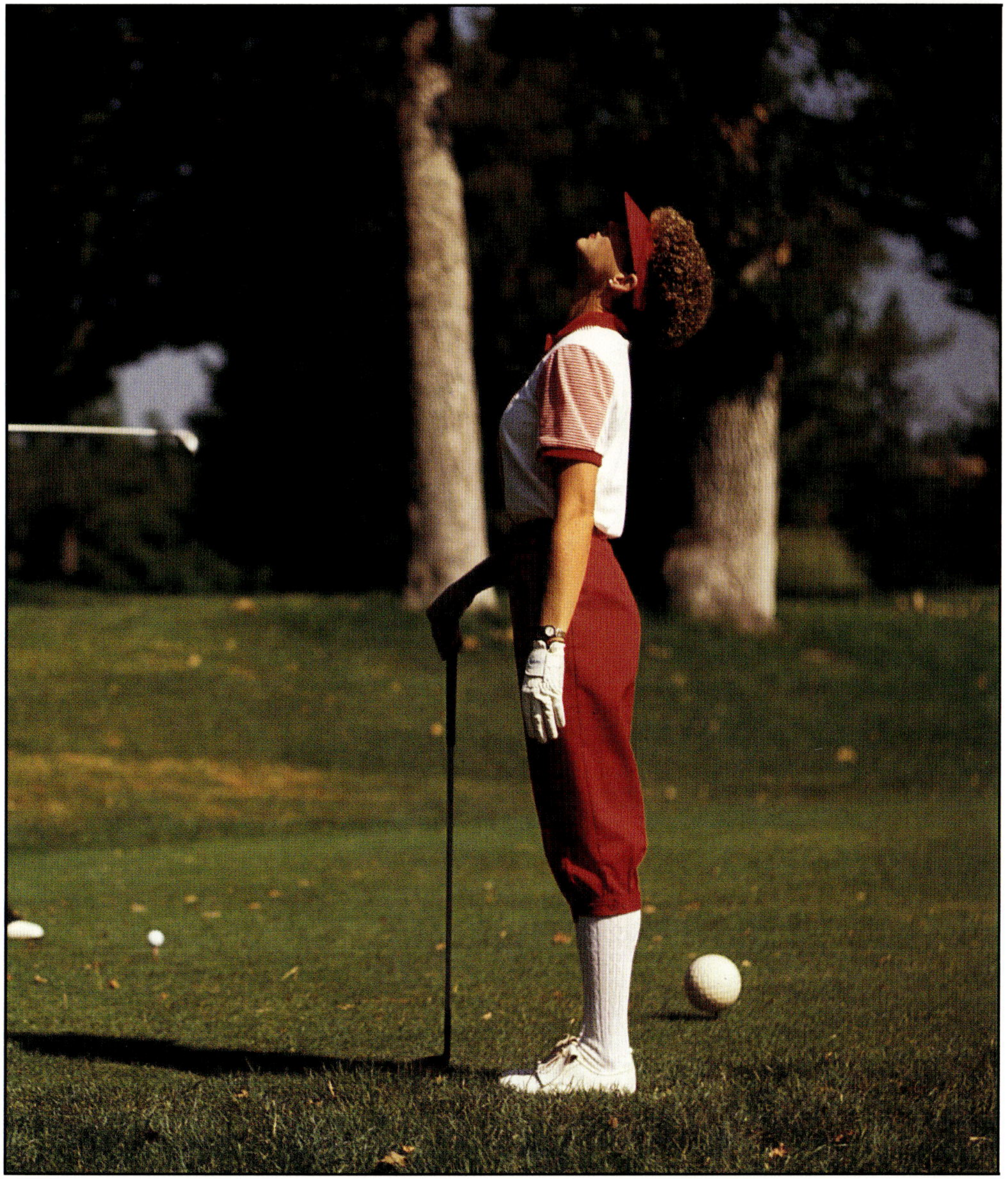

While standing upright, look up. Begin very gently with this exercise and hold up to 5 seconds to start with.

NECK STRETCH - Sides

While standing upright, turn head sideways to the left as far as comfortable. Repeat to right side.

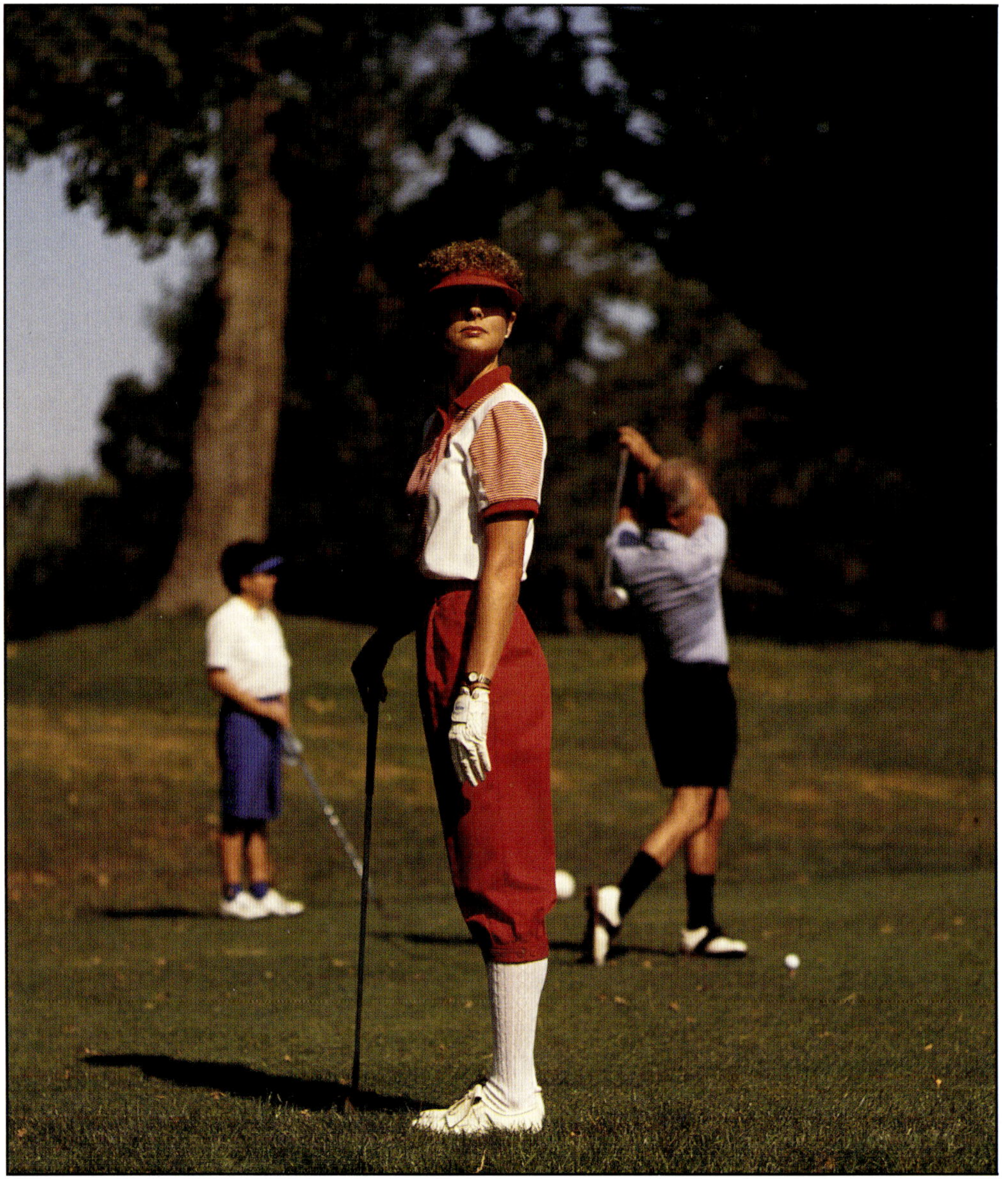

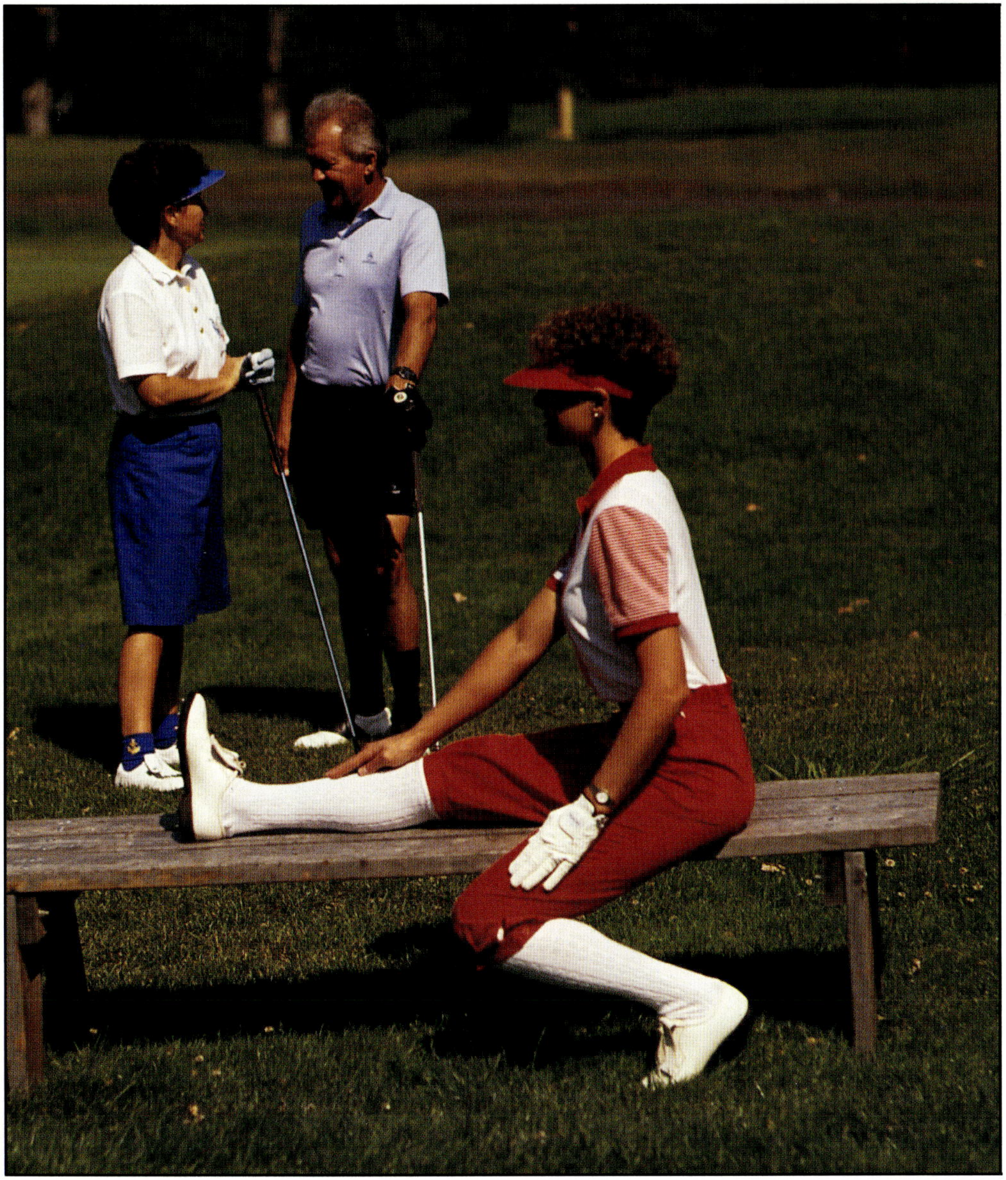

While sitting on a bench, fully extend leg along its length. Bend body forward from the hip toward fully extended leg. Feel stretch at back of thigh. Repeat stretch other side.

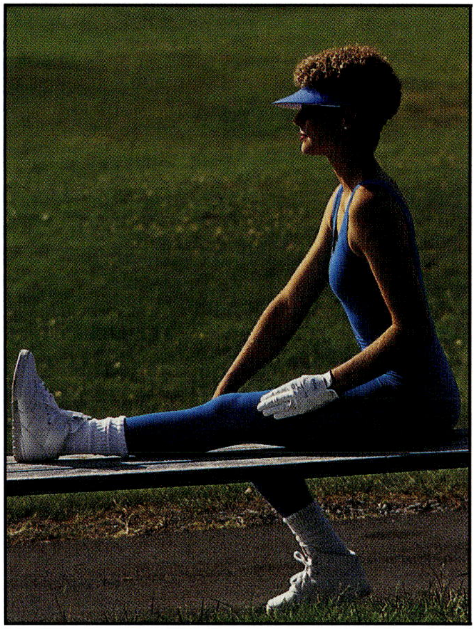

HAMSTRING STRETCH - Alternate

While standing upright, set your right heel up on stair. First stair is fine if you can feel a stretch in the back of your thigh. If not, place heel on the second or third stair or whatever until you feel a gentle stretch in the back of your right thigh. As you feel the tension subside bend body forward from the hip toward fully extended right leg until a comfortable stretch is felt. Avoid rounding your back. Repeat stretch other side.

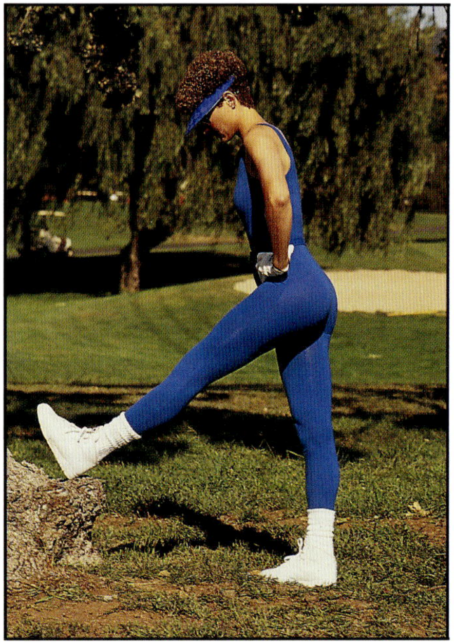

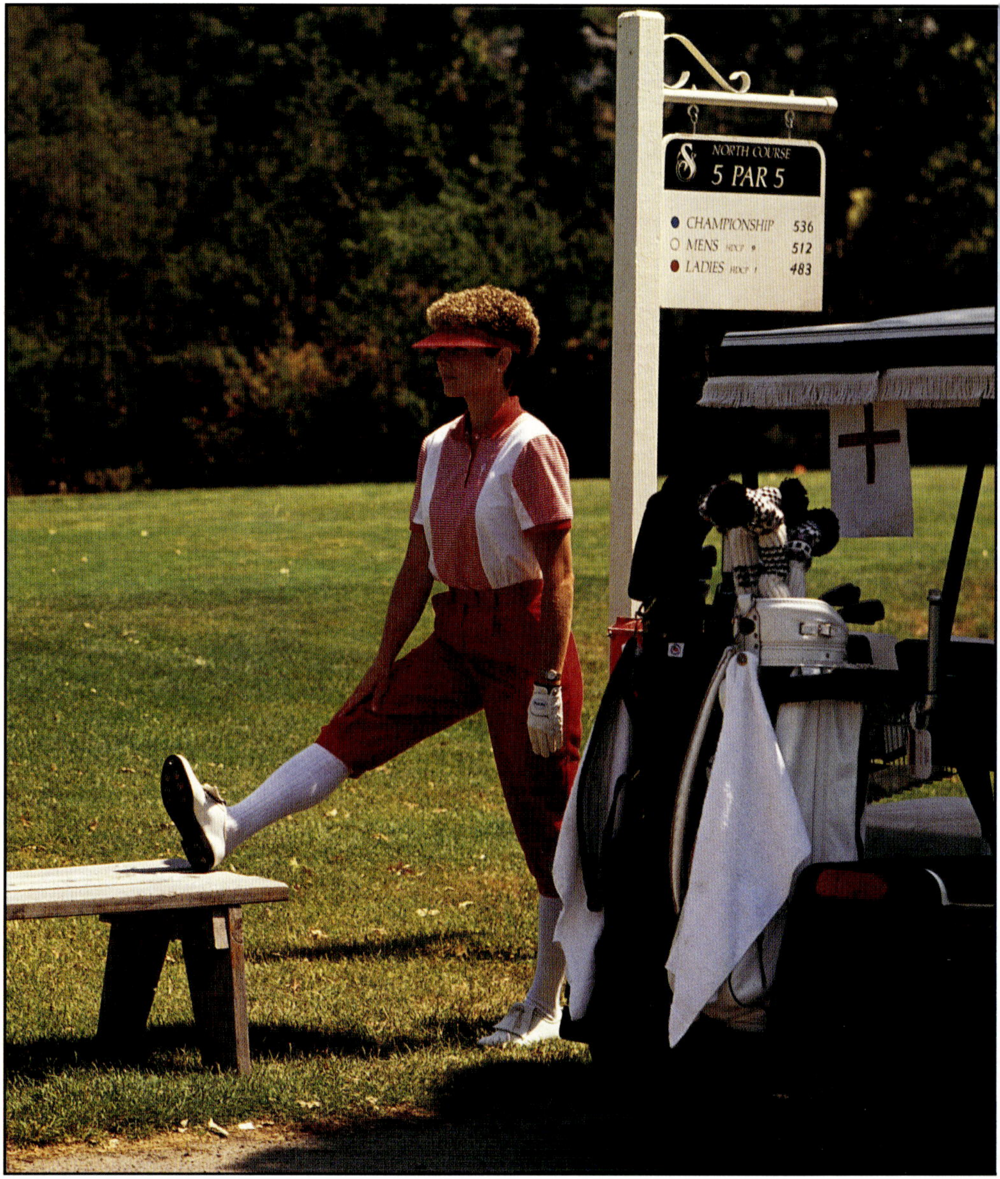

HAMSTRING STRETCH - Alternate

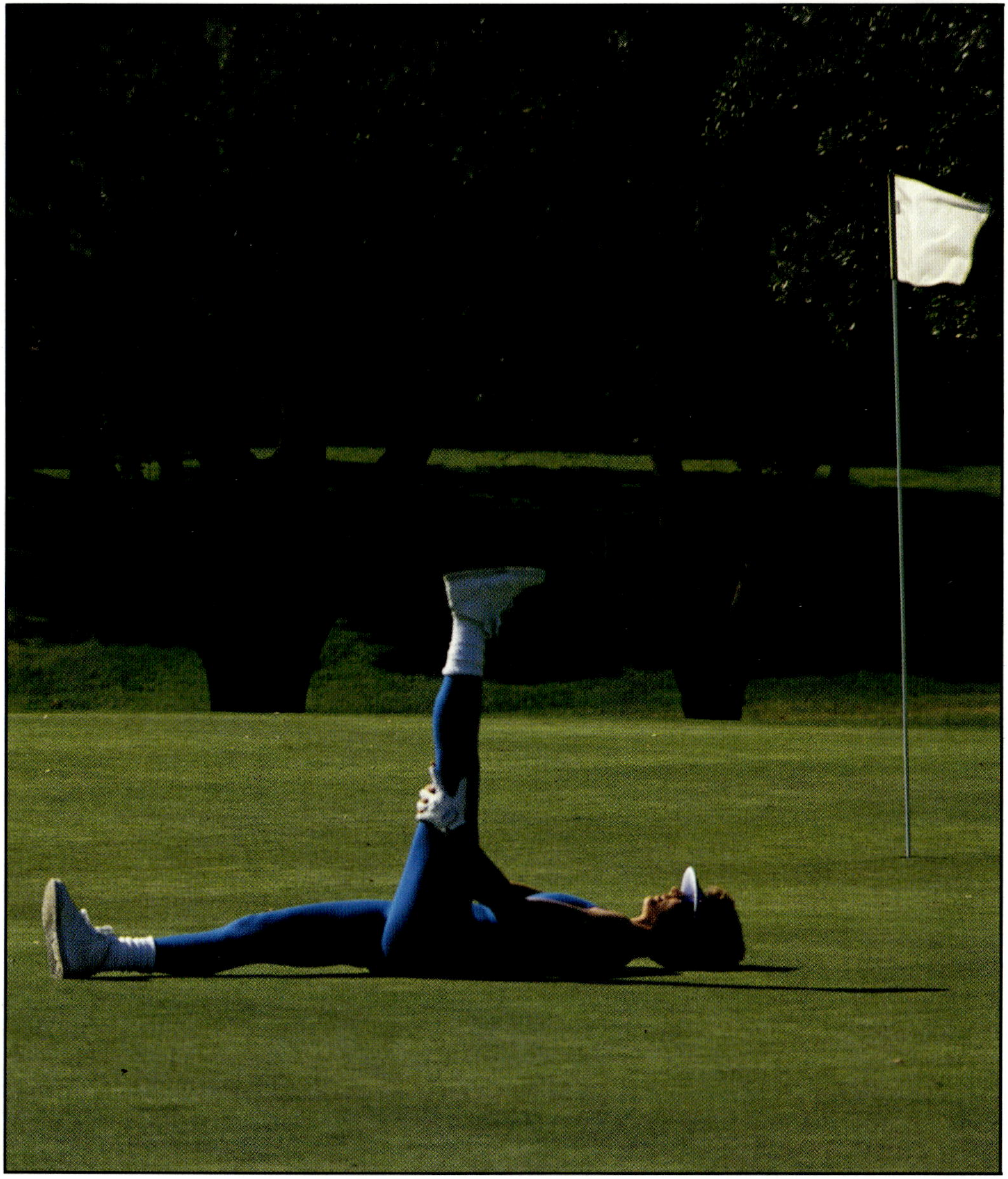

An alternate stretch is to lie down and fully extend your body. Bring your leg up and press your heel toward the sky. You may have your knee bent slightly. Feel stretch at back of thigh. Place your hands around thigh for support. Repeat stretch on other side.

CALF STRETCH

While resting hands on wall, tree or post, press right heel out and down and keep on ground. Point right toe toward the tree. Right leg is in straight line with the spine. Bend the left knee for stability. Repeat 2 times each side.

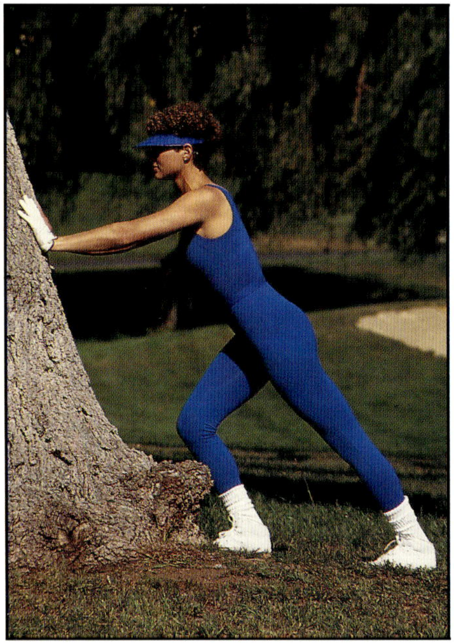

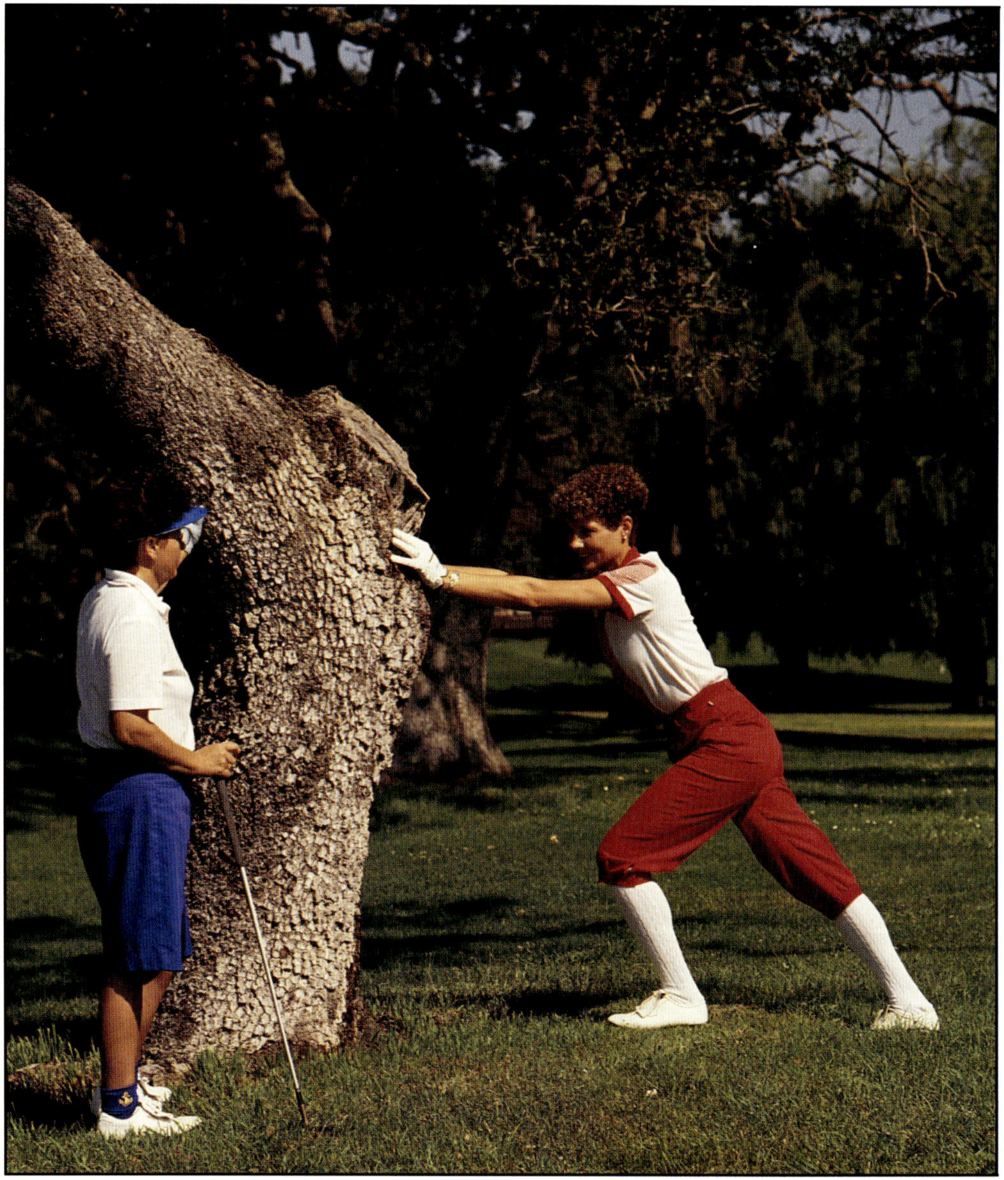

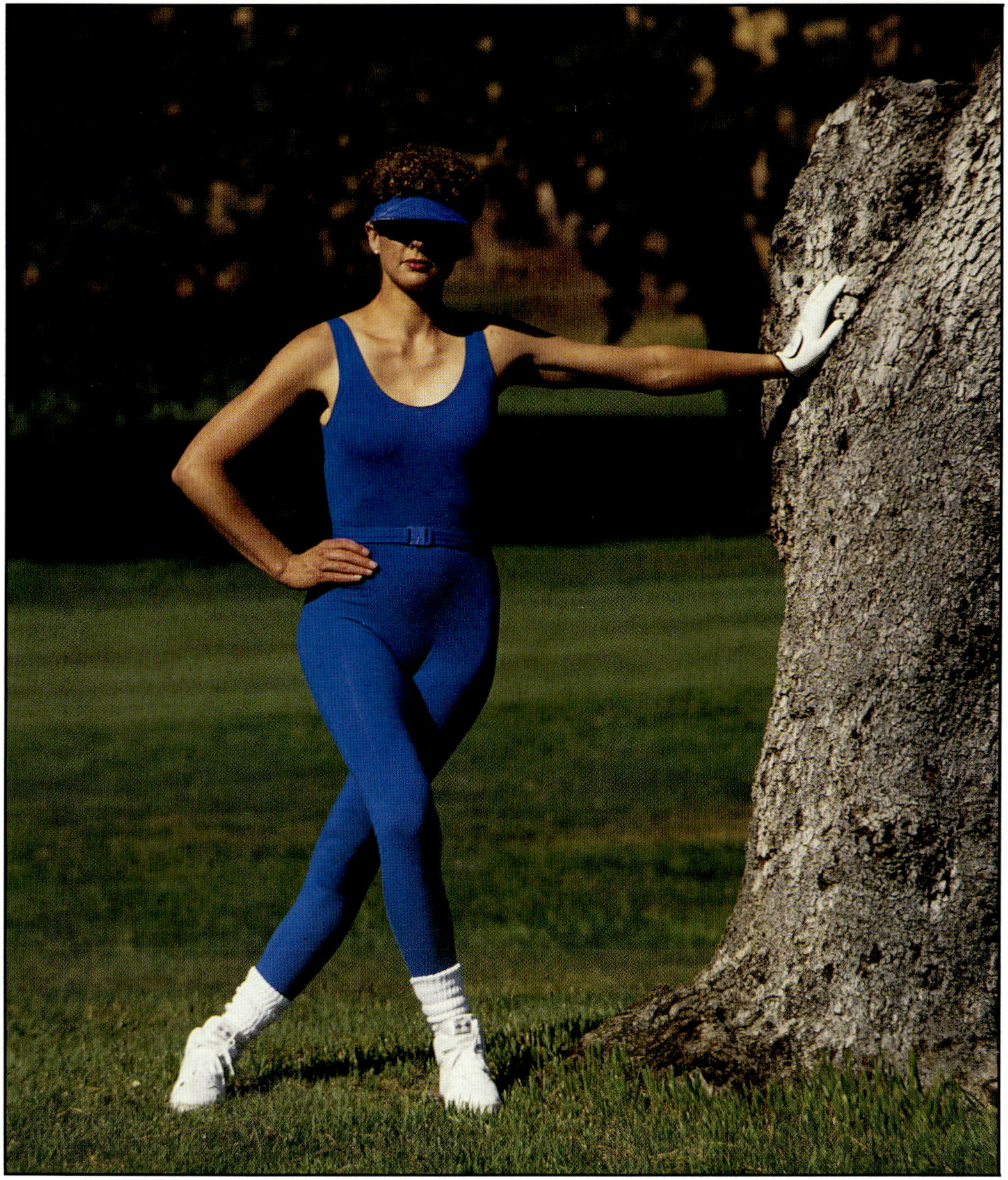

While standing upright, extend your left leg behind your right leg and out to the right slightly. Gently lean your left hip toward the tree to feel the stretch in the side of your hip. Steady your balance with your left hand on the tree. Repeat 2 times each side.

THIGH STRETCH - Easy

While standing erect on your left leg, bend your right knee and support your right foot and/or lower leg on a cart, bench — it will depend on your flexibility and what is available. To begin with, the object you choose need not be any higher than your knee. Be sure to tighten your stomach and buttock muscles in order to prevent your back from arching; and to increase the stretch. You should feel a gentle stretch in the front of your thigh. Repeat on each side 2 times.

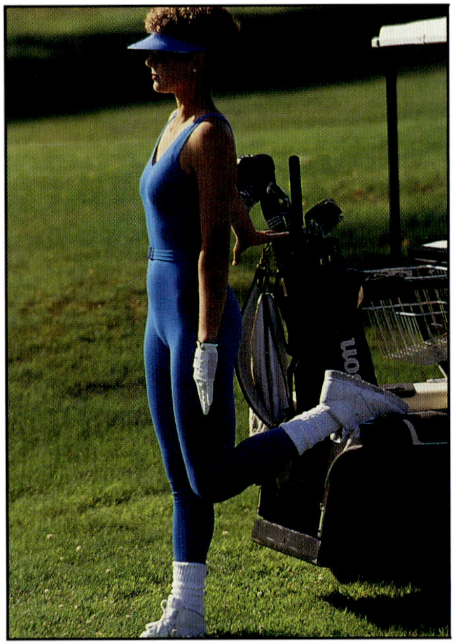

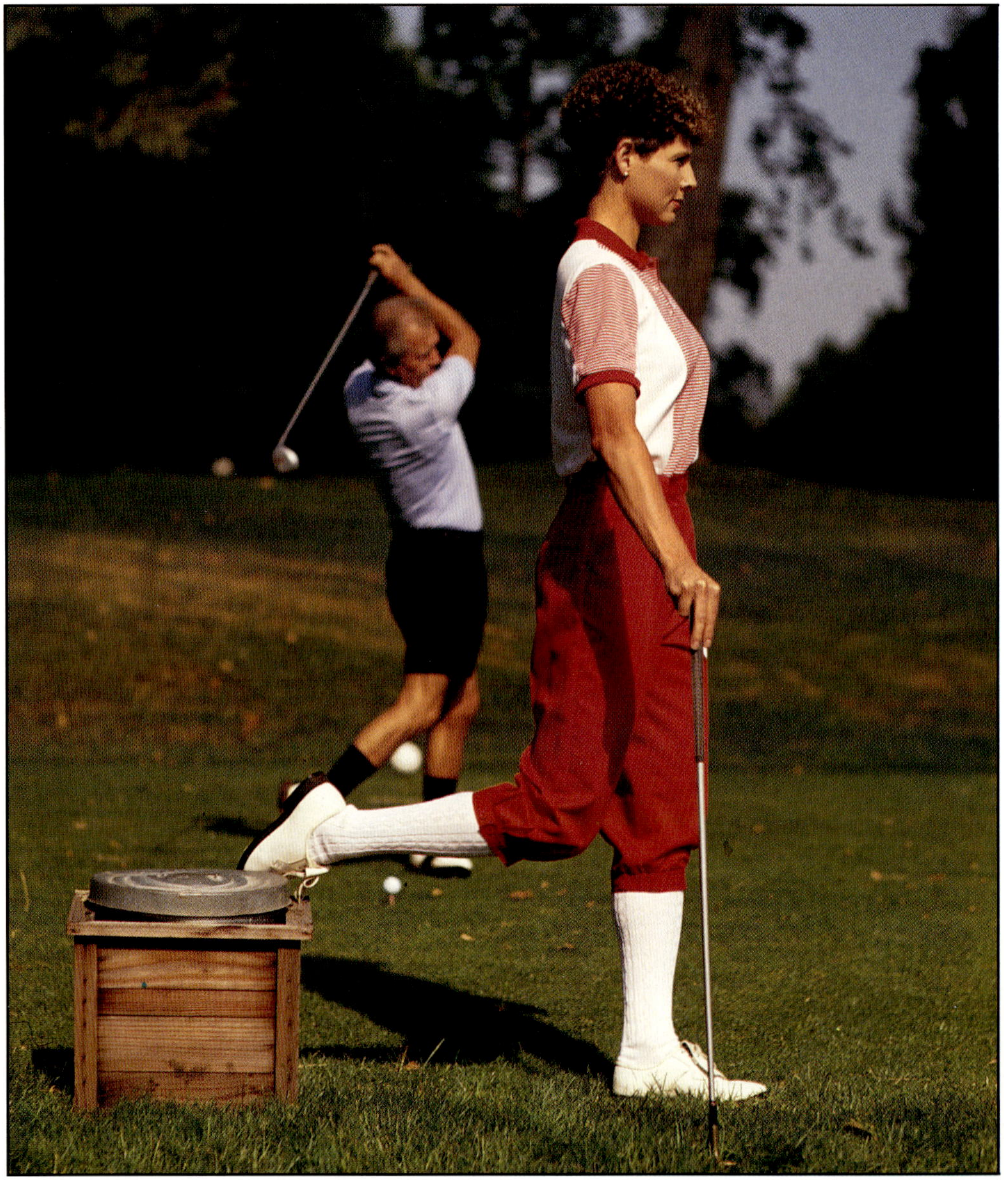

THIGH STRETCH - Advanced

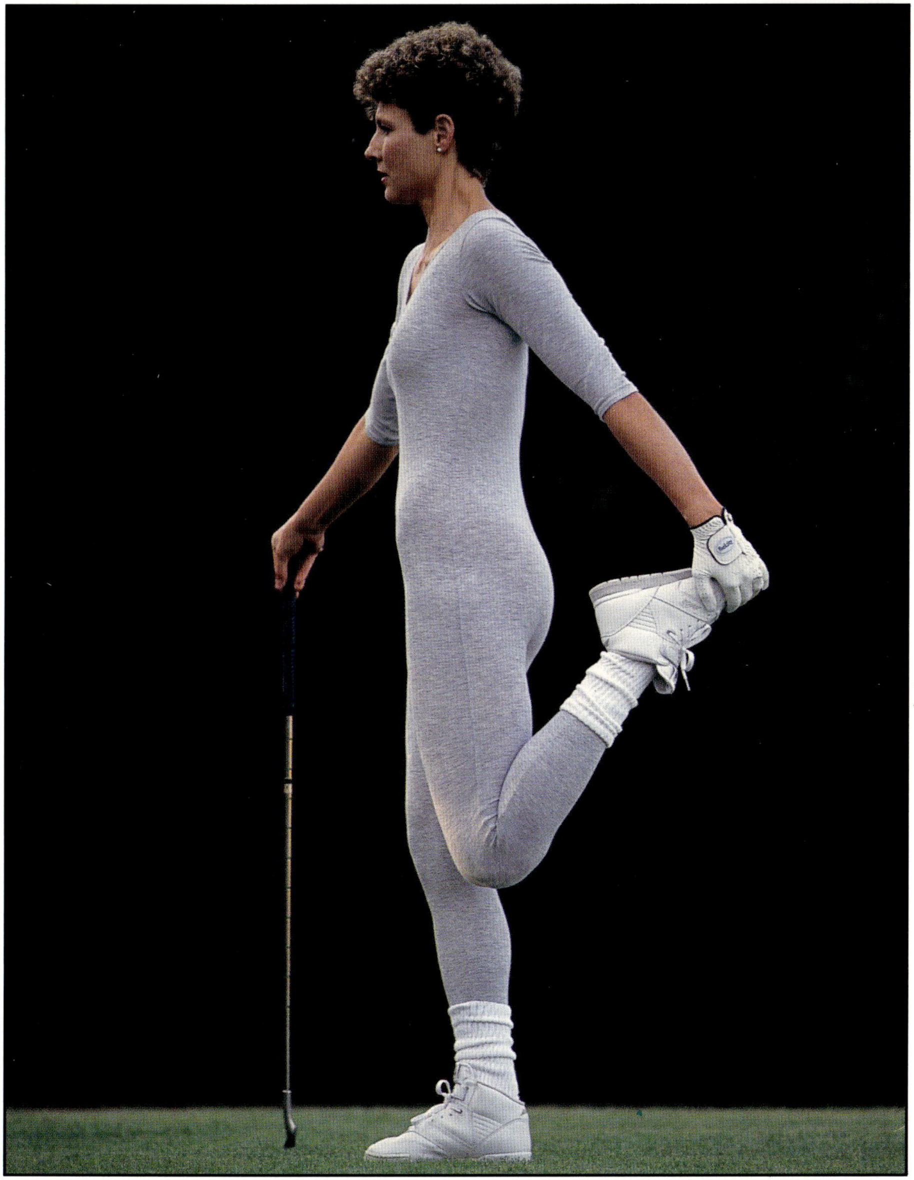

While standing erect on your right leg, bend your left knee and grasp your ankle with your left hand. Be sure to tighten your stomach and buttock muscles in order to prevent your back from arching. You should feel a gentle stretch in the front of your thigh. Repeat each side.

Palm out
Extend arm out in front with palm out. Pull palm with opposite hand toward your body in order to gently stretch the front of the hand, wrist, forearm and elbow. Repeat 2 times on each side.

Palm in
Extend arm out in front with palm in. Pull back of hand with opposite hand toward your body in order to gently stretch the back of the hand, wrist, forearm and elbow. Repeat 2 times on each side.

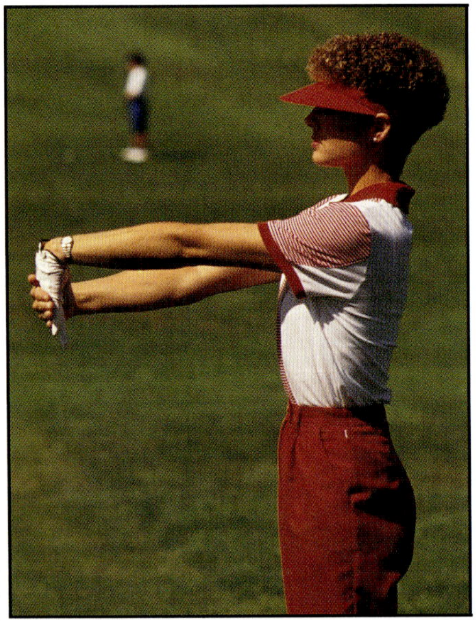

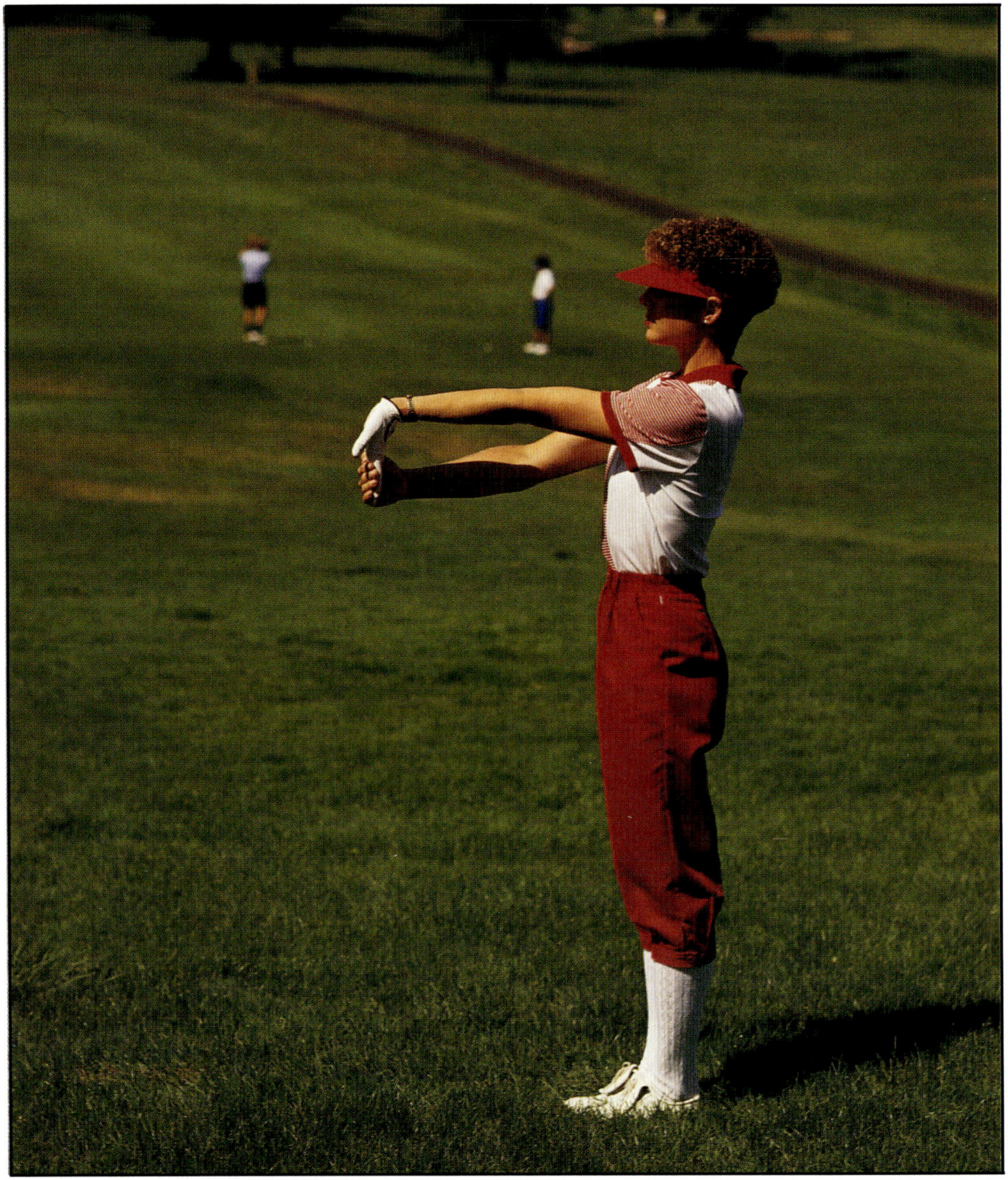

HALF SWING WARM UP

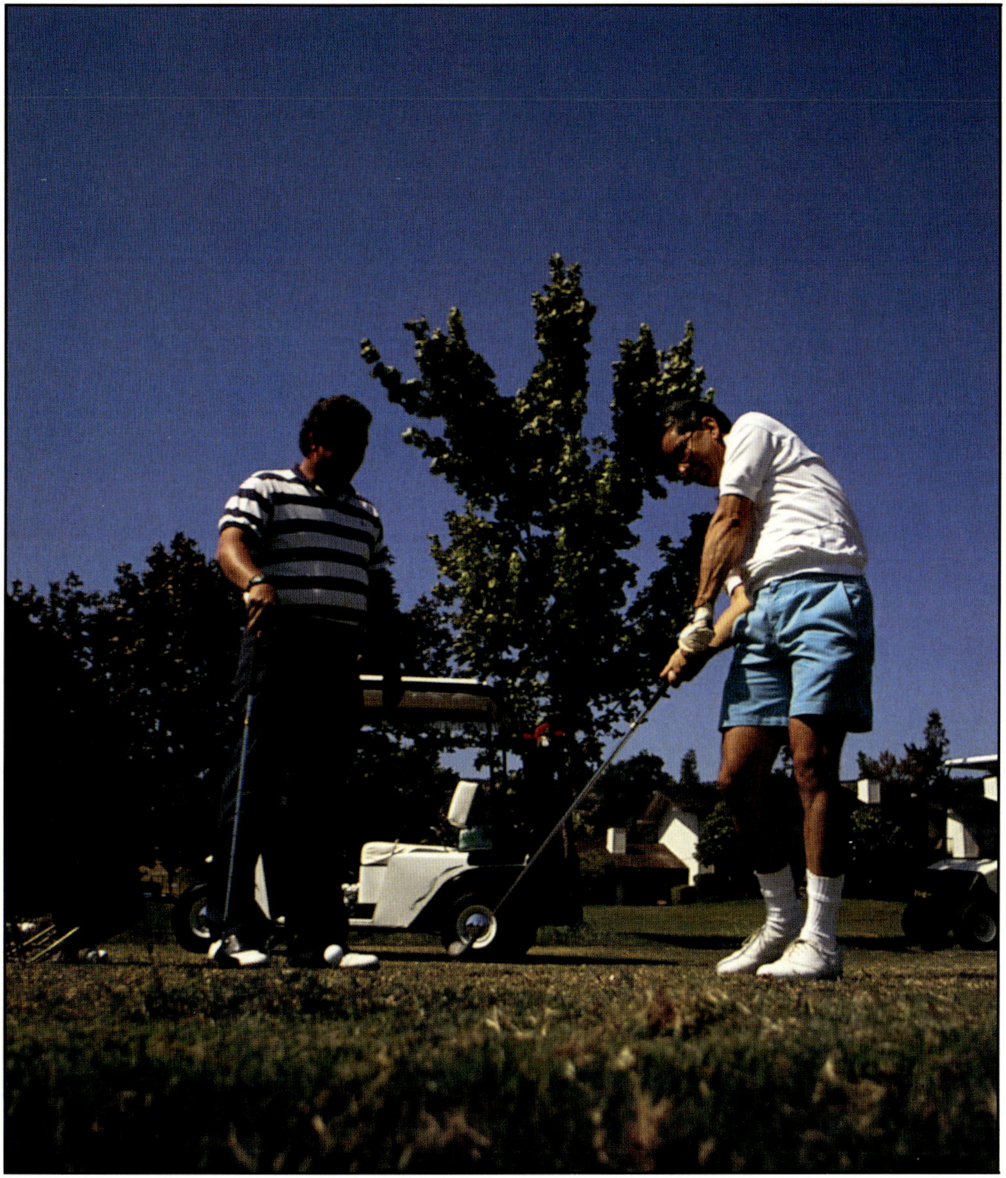

Now you are ready to do some half swing warm-ups using several clubs at once and then on to the driving range to hit a few balls.

If you begin to tighten up at any time, do a few of your favorite stretches. When you are in good condition and properly warmed up you are more likely to have a balanced coil, a clean follow through and you are more likely to putt well. Proper FOREPLAY can make all the difference in the world.

Drink plenty of water and remember to breathe deeply taking air all the way down into the bottom of your lungs.

Enjoy yourself and may the golfing gods be good to you!

SUGGESTED READING

FOREPLAY presents stretching for golf in the simplest format possible. We used this format because most of us are already overwhelmed by information. Also, the available time during the day for additional tasks is vanishing. If you would like to learn more, the following list of books will provide you with a good foundation. These are by no means the only books or videos available and you can find many more at your library or bookstore. Please feel free to write to us if you have added suggestions that would complement this list.

Hochschuler, M.D., Stephen. *Back in Shape.*
Boston: Houghton Mifflin Co., 1991

Ballard, Jimmy. *How to Perfect Your Golf Swing.*
Trumbull: Golf Digest/Tennis Inc., 1981

Wiren, Ph.D., Gary. *The PGA Manual of Golf.*
New York: Macmillan Publishing Company, 1991

Jobe, M.D., Frank. *30 Exercises for Better Golf.*
Inglewood: Champion Press, 1986

Hogan, Ben. *Five Lessons - The Modern Fundamentals of Golf.*
New York: Simon & Schuster, Inc.